Penguin Education

Penguin Science of Behaviour
General Editor: B. M. Foss

Abnormal and Clinical Psychology
Editors: Max Hamilton and Graham A. Foulds

An Introduction to Social Psychiatry
Ransom J. Arthur

Penguin Science of Behaviour
General Editor: B. M. Foss
Professor of Psychology, Bedford College,
University of London

Abnormal and Clinical
Psychology
Editors: Max Hamilton
Nuffield Professor of Psychiatry,
University of Leeds
Graham A. Foulds
University Department of
Psychiatry, Royal Edinburgh
Hospital

Cognitive Psychology
Editors: P. C. Dodwell
Professor of Psychology,
Queen's University at
Hamilton, Ontario
Anne Treisman
Institute of Experimental
Psychology, University of
Oxford

Developmental Psychology
Editor: B. M. Foss
Professor of Psychology,
Bedford College,
University of London

Industrial Psychology
Editor: Peter B. Warr
Assistant Director of the
Medical Research Council
Social and Applied Psychology
Unit, University of Sheffield

Method and History
Editor: W. M. O'Neil
Deputy Vice-Chancellor,
University of Sydney

Motivation and Emotion
Editors: Dalbir Bindra
Professor of Psychology,
McGill University, Montreal
Jane Stewart
Associate Professor of
Psychology, Sir George
Williams University, Montreal

Physiological Psychology
Editor: K. H. Pribram
Research Professor of
Psychology and Psychiatry,
Stanford University

Skills and Learning
Editor: Harry Kay
Professor of Psychology,
University of Sheffield

Social Psychology
Editor: Michael Argyle
Institute of Experimental
Psychology, University of
Oxford

An Introduction to Social Psychiatry

Ransom J. Arthur

Penguin Books

Penguin Books Ltd, Harmondsworth,
Middlesex, England
Penguin Books Inc., 7110 Ambassador Road,
Baltimore, Md 21207, U.S.A.
Penguin Books Australia Ltd,
Ringwood, Victoria, Australia

First published 1971
Copyright © Ransom J. Arthur, 1971

Made and printed in Great Britain by
Hazell Watson & Viney Ltd,
Aylesbury, Bucks
Set in Monotype Times

This book is sold subject to the condition that
it shall not, by way of trade or otherwise, be lent,
re-sold, hired out, or otherwise circulated without
the publisher's prior consent in any form of
binding or cover other than that in which it is
published and without a similar condition
including this condition being imposed on the
subsequent purchaser

Penguin Science of Behaviour

This book is one of an ambitious project, the Penguin Science of Behaviour, which covers a very wide range of psychological inquiry. Many of the short 'unit' texts are on central teaching topics, while others deal with present theoretical and empirical work which the Editors consider to be important new contributions to psychology. We have kept in mind both the teaching divisions of psychology and also the needs of psychology at work. For readers working with children, for example, some of the units in the field of Developmental Psychology will deal with psychological techniques in testing children, other units will deal with work on cognitive growth. For academic psychologists, there will be units in well-established areas such as Learning and Perception, but also units which do not fall neatly under any one heading, or which are thought of as 'applied', but which nevertheless are highly relevant to psychology as a whole.

The project is published in short units for two main reasons. Firstly, a large range of short texts at inexpensive prices gives the teacher a flexibility in planning his course and recommending texts for it. Secondly, the pace at which important new work is published requires the project to be adaptable. Our plan allows a unit to be revised or a fresh unit to be added with maximum speed and minimal cost to the reader.

Above, all, for students, the different viewpoints of many authors, sometimes overlapping, sometimes in contradiction, and the range of topics Editors have selected will reveal the complexity and diversity which exist beyond the necessarily conventional headings of an introductory course.

B.M.F.

Contents

	Editorial Foreword	9
1	Introduction	11
2	The Concept of Mental Illness	26
3	The Epidemiology of Mental Illness	39
4	Social Class and Psychiatric Disorder	63
5	Social Factors in the Onset of Disease	84
6	Transcultural Psychiatry	100
7	Social Psychiatry in the Hospital Setting	115
8	Community Psychiatry	130
9	Conclusion	146
	References	157
	Index	163

Editorial Foreword

It is now accepted as platitudinous that the society in which we live largely determines our behaviour. Given certain fundamental biological needs which our behaviour is intended to serve, the 'style' in which these needs are satisfied is determined by the influence of social interrelationships. The principle can be extended from normal to aberrant behaviour, which includes 'mental disorder' among other things. It is unfortunate that so many who write and speak on the subject go no further than this empty generalization. This is a great pity, for it gives the impression that the subject of social psychiatry is vague and nebulous.

Research in social psychiatry, as in other social sciences, suffers from the great difficulty of applying experimental methods. It therefore has to rely very much on other techniques for obtaining data on which to base theoretical generalizations. This book demonstrates that there has been real progress in this respect and gives a clear and detailed account of recent research. Captain Arthur starts by boldly tackling the controversy between the medical concept of 'mental disease' and the sociological concept of 'aberrant behaviour'. From here he moves on to consider epidemiological studies and especially social factors in the development of mental illness. In this section he gives an introduction to the new 'ecological' approach, to which he himself has made important contributions, to mental and psychosomatic disorders. From this, it is a natural step to consider transcultural psychiatry. Here he finds his position between the two extremist opinions, not by argument and theoretical presuppositions, but by basing himself firmly on empirical data.

Next, concerning himself with very different aspects of

social psychiatry, he gives an account of work done on the mental hospitals as a social institution and as a field of interpersonal relationships. The last chapter is concerned with the topical theme of community psychiatry.

Captain Aurthur's style of writing is clear, economical and free from vague, diffuse jargon. The deceptive ease with which the text can be read hides the art that has gone into the short, yet thorough, exposition.

M.H.

1 Introduction

Diseases, like wealth, are unequally distributed amongst mankind. The old have degenerative arthritis, the young measles and chickenpox. Sickle cell anaemia is common amongst Africans but rare in Europe. Cancer of the skin is frequently seen in Ireland but seldom encountered in Africa. Cancer of the breast, although not unknown in men, occurs with very much less frequency than it does in women. Silicosis is a disease of overburdened miners while coronary heart disease predominates in the well-fed and sedentary members of affluent, developed societies.

Even within relatively homogeneous groups diseases strike some members more than others. For example, Hinkle, Plummer and Whitney (1961) described a group of employees of a telephone company in an eastern region of the United States of America. Ten per cent of this group had a risk of becoming ill that was at least double that for the group as a whole, and the 10 per cent of individuals who were prone to illness accounted for 34 per cent of the total disability of the entire group. Their illness distribution was in marked contrast to that of the healthiest 10 per cent of the group, who experienced only 1 per cent of the overall morbidity. The phenomenon of disease clustering in certain individuals held true for both major and minor illnesses.

A similar study of illness patterns in the crew of a naval cruiser found that 25 per cent of the men developed over 50 per cent of the illnesses noted by the medical department during a six-month cruise. Amongst those who had the greatest number of illness episodes, there was a distinct trend toward a greater variety of illnesses than amongst the other, less susceptible members of the group. Thus, they did not simply have repetitions of the same illnesses, but rather seemed to be vulnerable to all kinds of illnesses involving many different organ systems and many different causations, including illnesses manifested by disturbances of mood, thought and behaviour. This observation has held true over all groups studied thus far. What is true for illness classified as physical or organic in nature seems also to apply to those phenomena which are called mental disorders, emotional illnesses or psychiatric diseases. These, too, occur with varying frequency in persons of differing age, sex, race, social class, dwelling place and circumstances.

In order to study scientifically variations in the rate of afflictions, one may utilize a systematic method of observation known as epidemiology which deals with the analysis of the distribution of diseases. Over the years epidemiology has been variously defined and (as one might infer from the name) epidemiological studies once dealt primarily with those catastrophic and epidemic infections of mankind such as the plague or typhoid fever. But now, in an era of mass sanitation and mass immunization, the interests of epidemiologists have moved towards the study of those chronic diseases which afflict the advanced nations of Western Europe and North America. Epidemiology might be defined as that science which deals with the distribution of diseases in space and time and the factors which account for these distributions. Epidemiologists try to find populations with differing rates of illness and then try to compare their respective environments in the hope of discovering possible causes of disease. They examine the conditions under which diseases flourish and under which they are extinguished. As a discipline, epidemiology leans heavily upon demography, statistics, clinical medicine and pathology. It owes to statistics and demography the mathematical techniques for delineating population characteristics, and to clinical medicine and pathology the definition of diseases and the conceptualization of pathological entities and processes. Morris (1957) of the Social Medicine Research Unit, London, has stated seven actual and potential uses of epidemiology.

First, *historical epidemiology*, the study of the history of the health of populations and of the historical trends of diseases and their accompanying changes in character. For example, syphilis, tuberculosis and streptococcal diseases were all clearly more lethal in the past than they are to our present relatively resistant populations. It may also be possible to make projections into the future from such historical studies of disease trends.

Second, the study of *community health*. Through epidemiology it is possible to measure the dimensions and distribution of sickness in terms of incidence, prevalence and mortality, to define health problems for community action and to assess their relative importance and priority, and to identify particularly vulnerable subsections of the population.

Third, the *operational analysis of health services*. Epidemiology may be part of an operational analysis of community health in terms of needs and demands. It can help define the standards and efficacy of services rendered and suggest how these might be improved, and furnish useful information to administrative authorities charged with the development of further community health programmes.

Fourth, *individual risks*. Epidemiology can, from the examination of large groups and cohorts of people, develop data which give the chances of individuals with certain characteristics developing a certain disorder within a specified period of time.

Fifth, *completion of the clinical picture*. Epidemiology can be of great aid to clinical medicine by developing a natural history of disorders. The relative numbers of patients having the disease in varying degrees of severity can be ascertained by means of longitudinal studies which follow the course of remission and relapse, detect early subclinical disease and discover pathological antecedents of the actual disorder. A common difficulty in clinical medicine is that the clinicians, often seeing just those severe cases which appear in hospital, have a biased picture of the range of combinations and permutations possible in any given disorder. A good example is rheumatoid arthritis. Clinical studies and clinical textbooks all point out what a serious and grave disease this is, involving many organs other than the joints, for example, the heart, the eyes, the gastro-intestinal system, skin, etc. But though this is very true of those people sick enough to require long-term hospitalization, epidemiological surveys in the community indicate that there are a great many people, in fact, the majority of sufferers from rheumatoid arthritis, who are able to continue their lives with only minor interruptions and with relatively minor treatment by such drugs as aspirin.

Sixth, the *identification of syndromes*. Epidemiology, by describing the distribution and degrees of association and dissociation of clinical phenomena in a population, may be able to indicate that certain characteristics of patients cluster together to form a distinct entity.

Finally, seventh, *analytic and experimental epidemiology*. Epidemiology may be used to search for the causes of disease by studying disease incidence in various groups and defining these groups in terms of their composition, their life experiences, their behaviour, their environment and their genetic constitution. In addition to this analytic work there may be deliberately planned or, occasionally, naturally occurring experiments in which one group of humans experience some environmental change while another group does not, and the consequences of change and no change may then be compared.

Lin and Standley (1962) feel that epidemiology is useful in the field of mental health in assessing the incidence and prevalence of different types of mental ill health in a population as a basis for the prevention, treatment and control of these disorders. It may uncover associations between population characteristics that clarify the origin of mental disorders and provide a test for etiological hypotheses originating from the laboratory or from clinical studies. It can assess the rate of spontaneous recovery against which the effectiveness of preventive and therapeutic measures can be evaluated.

There are two fundamental definitions of disease frequency which are essential to the understanding of any epidemiological statement. The first term is *prevalence*. The prevalence of the disease is its frequency at a given moment or period of time. If it is of a given moment it is called a point prevalence;

if of some length of time it is a period prevalence. Prevalence is a measure of what exists or prevails and is expressed as a proportion of the population who exhibits a disease at a particular instant. For example, all those residents of Plymouth who have diphtheria on 1 January 1968 is a statement of point prevalence and can be expressed as a rate: the number of diphtheritics per 1000 population as of 1 January 1968. The other term of fundamental importance is *incidence*, which is defined as the number of new cases of a disease that come into recognized being during a specified period in a specified unit of population. For example, all new cases of diphtheria which occurred in Plymouth during the calendar year 1968 is a statement of incidence and is expressed as a rate: the number of new cases per 1000 inhabitants of Plymouth during 1968. Incidence rates have been called the fundamental measurement of epidemiology; but they depend upon a precise knowledge of disease onset, often difficult to ascertain, and of the membership of the population 'at risk', a factor which is affected by migration. Both incidence and point prevalence are affected by the arbitrariness of much case finding. Point prevalence (hereafter simply called prevalence) is determined by an interplay of dynamic forces, one of which is incidence. The other forces have to do with the removal of cases. Removal from the register of illness may be due to the patient's recovery, to his death or to his emigration from the subject population.

Although the beginnings of epidemiology might well be traced back to the ancient world and to the great physician Hippocrates, certainly the major impetus to its development as a science in the modern era came from two seventeenth-century Englishmen, Graunt and Petty, both from Hampshire. John Graunt was a man of many parts – a mercer, a music teacher, a captain and later major of militia, and a Fellow of the Royal Society. He was the first to analyse figures relating to birth and death as shown by the Bills of Mortality compiled by the clergy of England. He demonstrated many perennial truths of demography including the excess of male over female births, the excess of urban deaths over rural ones for any given age group, and the high mortality then prevalent in young children. Sir William Petty, a physician, Vice-Principal of Brasenose College, Oxford, and Professor of Anatomy, made important proposals for the formation of the equivalent of a General Registry Office or central statistical department to compile statistical information related to the mortality and morbidity of the entire national population. He also suggested the principle of the life or survivorship table, depicting the systematic erosion by selective mortality of a cohort of individuals born at the same time. The epidemiological outlook, depending as it does upon painstaking induction guided by working hypotheses, is very congenial to the British philosophical tradition of empiricism exemplified by the work of such men as Berkeley, Locke and Hume.

The classical example of epidemiological research still remains the meticulous and dedicated study of Asiatic cholera made by Dr John Snow (Richardson and Hampton Frost, 1936) in London in the nineteenth century. The parallel here with the epidemiology of mental disorder is exceedingly apt, because when Snow studied cholera, its cause, as with many mental disorders today, was uncertain.

Cholera is a loathsome disease caused as we now know by infection with an organism known as the vibrio cholerae. The vibrio enters the human intestinal tract when the individual ingests some contaminated material, usually water contaminated by sewage containing infected human excrement. The disease is characterized by an abrupt and fulminating course with the passage of immense amounts of fluid from the intestinal tract to such a degree that the patient becomes dehydrated and drained of minerals and suffers circulatory collapse. It struck Great Britain in the nineteenth century; there were severe epidemics in 1832, 1849 and 1854. The epidemic of 1854 swept Oxford with special severity and a chill note of dread penetrated even the walls of the most ancient of Oxford colleges. There were many theories current then about the cause of cholera. For example, Dr Ackland, in his *Memoir on the Cholera at Oxford in the Year 1854*, showed that the worst hit parts of the city were in the low-lying areas, and he suggested that the disorder was caused by the bad air coming from marshy soil. There were many other etiological theories advanced which seemed perfectly reasonable at the time but which in the light of current knowledge now seem merely fanciful.

Snow, himself, was a man of some interest. He, like Captain Cook, the famous explorer of the South Seas, was born the son of a humble Yorkshire farmer. (Social mobility is not exclusively a feature of the twentieth century. Indeed, we will examine later the role it has played in the incidence of mental disorders themselves.) He qualified as a physician and then, as have so many famous Englishmen, Scots, Welshmen and Irishmen, went to London to seek his fortune. He became a prominent physician and had the honour of attending Queen Victoria on the occasion of the births of Prince Leopold and Princess Beatrice, when he was employed as the anaesthetist using a chloroform soaked handkerchief as the instrument of anesthesia. Although he had a flourishing practice he found time to carry out extensive research projects essentially on his own, both in terms of finances and actual field work. In speaking of the second edition of his monumental work, *On the Mode of Communication of Cholera*, he said that he had spent in developing the data on which the book was based more than two hundred pounds in hard cash, and he had realized in return scarcely so many shillings. Snow had witnessed the cholera epidemic of 1832 in Newcastle as well as the epidemic of 1846 in London. As a result of his observations he formulated the hypothesis that the frequency of cholera in the various geographic areas of London was related to the water supply of the respective districts. He hypothesized further that water supplied to certain districts contained some noxious pollutant or effluvium which in some way was causing the disorder. One must remember that this was some years prior to the formulation of the germ theory of disease and thirty years prior to the demonstrations of the actual cholera organism by Koch. Snow noted that those districts supplied by the water of the Southwark and Vauxhall Company, which drew its water straight from the Thames by the Battersea Fields half a mile north of Vauxhall Bridge, had a very high rate of cholera

Table 1 Deaths from Cholera in London Sub-Districts in 1853

	Population in 1851	Deaths from cholera in 1853	Deaths from cholera in each 100,000 living	Water supply
St Saviour, Southwark	19,709	45	227	
St Olave	8015	19	237	
St John, Horsleydown	11,360	7	61	
St James, Bermondsey	18,899	21	111	
St Mary Magdalen	13,934	27	193	
Leather Market	15,295	23	153	Southwark and
Rotherhithe*	17,805	20	112	Vauxhall Water
Wandsworth	9611	3	31	Company only
Battersea	10,560	11	104	
Putney	5280	—	—	
Camberwell	17,742	9	50	
Peckham	19,444	7	36	
Christchurch, Southwark	16,022	7	43	
Kent Road	18,126	37	204	
Borough Road	15,862	26	163	
London Road	17,836	9	50	
Trinity, Newington	20,922	11	52	

St Peter, Walworth	29,861	23	77	Lambeth Water Company and Southwark and Vauxhall Company
St Mary, Newington	14,033	5	35	
Waterloo (1st part)	14,088	1	7	
Waterloo (2nd part)	18,348	7	38	
Lambeth Church (1st part)	18,409	9	48	
Lambeth Church (2nd part)	26,784	11	41	
Kennington (1st part)	24,261	12	49	
Kennington (2nd part)	18,848	6	31	
Brixton	14,610	2	13	
Clapham	16,290	10	61	
St George, Camberwell	15,849	6	37	
Norwood	3977	—	—	Lambeth Water Company only
Streatham	9023	—	—	
Dulwich	1632	—	—	
First 12 subdistricts	167,654	192	114	Southwark and Vauxhall
Next 16 subdistricts	301,149	182	60	Both Companies
Last 3 subdistricts	14,632	—	—	Lambeth Company

* A part of Rotherhithe was supplied by the Kent Water Company; but there was no cholera in this part.

Source: Snow (see Richardson and Hampton Frost, 1936, p. 73)

mortality, both in 1849 and in 1854. On the other hand, those districts served by the Lambeth Water Company, which drew water upstream near Thames Ditton, had a death rate very much lower than those districts exclusively supplied by the Southwark and Vauxhall Company.

Those districts in which there was an intermixture of houses, some served by the Southwark and Vauxhall Company and some by the Lambeth Company, had a mortality rate intermediate between those districts served by one company alone. These observations gave great weight to his hypothesis that some substance in polluted drinking water was responsible for the onset of cholera. Further corroborative evidence was furnished by the exceedingly high rate of cholera amongst sailors and dock workers who drank water obtained by simply dropping a bucket in the Thames and pulling the water straight out and drinking it without any further processing. However, there might have been many factors other than the water supply in which these districts differed. For example, the districts supplied by one company might have represented districts of high social class, with good nutrition and good medical attention, whereas the other company might have supplied working-class districts. Therefore, it was essential for Dr Snow to examine those districts in which houses existed side by side, where there were dwellings similar in type and housing people of similar occupations and social class, differing only in that one house had its water supplied by the Lambeth Company and its neighbour by the Southwark and Vauxhall. He conducted a field examination in the various subdistricts of Lambeth, Southwark and Newington where houses by one or another of the two water companies were intermixed. There was a good deal of difficulty in obtaining even such simple information as to which water company supplied a given house. Often the residents could not remember the name of the water company and had to check their receipts. In the case of working people who paid weekly rents, the rates were very often paid by someone else, and the residents did not know from which company their water came. However, Dr Snow solved this difficulty by inventing a chemical test to distinguish the Lambeth water from that of Southwark and Vauxhall. As he said, 'It would, indeed, have been almost impossible for me to complete the inquiry, if I had not found that I could distinguish the water of the two companies with perfect certainty by a chemical test' (Richardson and Hampton Frost, 1936, pp. 77–8). This test determined the amount of sodium chloride in the water, and because the supplies of the two companies were drawn from differing sources on the tidal Thames, they were found to be clearly distinguishable in this

Table 2 Deaths from Cholera in London in 1854

	Number of houses	Deaths from cholera	Death in each 10,000 houses
Southwark and Vauxhall Company	40,046	1263	315
Lambeth Company	26,107	98	37
Rest of London	256,423	1422	59

Source: Richardson and Hampton Frost (1936, p. 86)

respect. Within areas supplied by both companies, the respective cholera death rates for the customers of each company were roughly the same as those of the customers in the area supplied exclusively by a given company. Furthermore, even though the majority of the Lambeth Company customers were located in areas primarily supplied by the Southwark and Vauxhall Company in which cholera was high prevalent, the death rate of these Lambeth Company people was no higher than that for the rest of London. Therefore, the hypothesis that the incidence and prevalence of cholera was related to the supply of polluted water was confirmed. This confirmation, however, did not establish final proof of the cause of cholera. This required the advancement of bacteriology and other sciences which could actually isolate the true etiological agent. Nevertheless, this type of field study and epidemiological reasoning did provide a strong inference as to the etiology of the disorder. We are, of course, treading on dangerous ground when speaking about a unitary cause of any given disease. Not only is the reality concerning disease often very complex, but also, as David Hume long ago pointed out, 'We are never able in a single instance to discover any power or necessary connection, any quality which binds the effect of the cause and renders the one infallible consequence of the other. We only find that one does actually, in fact, follow the other.' In other words, the inference underlying our thoughts on causation is that the future will be like the past and having observed in the past that 'b' inevitably follows 'a' we conceptualize the phenomenon as one of causation and necessary consequence. Certainly our thinking on disease causation follows this inferential pattern.

Dr Snow's researches show how a model epidemiological investigation proceeds. First, by means of observation and what might be termed descriptive epidemiology, the differential prevalence of a given disease is noted. Then an hypothesis is formulated about environmental factors which might account for this differential prevalence. This step might be termed analytic epidemiology. Finally, painstaking field work is carried out, preferably utilizing an instrument which can accurately identify that environmental factor in which one is most interested. In Dr Snow's case this was the chemical test for chlorides which identified the presumably polluted water. The population at risk within the various districts had to be accurately specified and, in turn, this depended upon an accurate census of the area's inhabitants. Maps showing clustering of cases were also illuminating. Basic, however, to the success of the entire investigation was the clear definition of a case. Cholera is such a dramatic disease and has so characteristic a course that there would be scarcely any quarrel as to the correct diagnosis of a case during an epidemic period. Alas, just the opposite condition prevails in the field of mental illness. In fact, some students of the field deny that there is even such an entity as psychiatric disease. To understand the problem of psychiatric diagnoses, however, some further discussion of the concept of disease and illness is necessary.

Disorders of bodily functioning exist throughout the animal kingdom and certainly did not spare early man. Bones from the Stone Age show evidence of infection, and Egyptian mummies still bear the preserved parasites which infested the body during life. But the ways in which men have conceptualized these phenomena have changed with the passage of time and civilizations. There appears to be a universal necessity for some intellectual structure to give meaning to life's events and among these disease is no exception. It has been variously viewed as a form of punishment for moral transgression, possession by evil spirits or the result of some malign forces in nature.

In ancient Greece, Plato saw health as a state of harmony and disease as a state of discord. Disease was defined in terms of unnatural excesses or deficiencies of the four constituents of the body – earth, fire, water and air. Health was seen by the Platonic School as a state of equilibrium between these elements, and when the balance was disrupted or impaired, illness resulted. In the works of Hippocrates there is what Riese (1953) has called the historical conception of disease; that is, the symptoms and signs exhibited by the patient are given meaning only in terms of their being manifestations of some greater entity, namely, the disease itself. Thus all the symptoms were viewed as being interrelated and were seen in an historical light. In fact, the first use of individual clinical histories appeared in the works of the Hippocratic School. The views of Galen, the great physician of Tome who lived in the second century, summarized the thinking of the ancient world on the problems of disease. He thought of disease in what might be called pathophysiological terms, however rudimentary and incorrect his physiology. Disease was viewed once again in terms of a dynamic interplay between four forces or humours: blood, mucus, black bile and yellow bile. It is, of course, necessary to have some kind of theoretical point of view into which one can order the innumerable and diverse observations made in the course of medical practice. As the medical historian, Henry Sigerist, pointed out (1958), 'Every theory is philosophical in its nature. It works with the thoughts, with the concepts, available at any particular epoch, thus moulding the culture of the time.'

With the rise of the study of anatomy during the Renaissance, diseases began to be viewed as disruptions of the structure of the human fabric. In the nineteenth century there dawned a Golden Age of studies of morbid anatomy, or pathology as it is now known. In Central Europe, Rudolph Virchow and Carl Freiherr Von Rokitansky performed tens of thousands of autopsies upon patients who had died of all manner of disease in the great hospitals of Germany and Austria. These scientists were able to correlate closely the symptoms and signs which the patients showed during life with the lesions or structural changes shown in the organs at necropsy. At the very time this patho-anatomical conception of disease was becoming increasingly dominant, the science of bacteriology was growing and the germ theory of infectious disease was born. At the same time more and more combinations of symptoms which appeared with a certain regularity together became identified as separate diseases; and an increasing number of these diseases seemed to have a unitary microbial cause. For a time the unitary etiological theory of disease seemed triumphant. For example, out of the old dustbin disease category of 'fever' used until the nineteenth century, there had emerged a whole series of recognized specific febrile diseases ranging from malaria to typhoid fever, all of which appeared to have a specific parasite as a cause: a bacterium in the case of typhoid fever and a protozoan in the case of malaria. But even during this era of a mechanistic view of illness, there were many voices raised in protest against the simplistic thinking apparent in this conception. In the first place, there appeared to be a number of impairments of health or deviations from the norm for which a specific microbial cause could not be found. In the second place, even in undoubtedly germ-caused diseases such as tuberculosis, it became clear that something more than merely the presence of the bacteria was necessary for clinical disease to develop. The individual who succumbed to tuberculosis seemed, in addition to exposure to the bacterium, to possess certain genetic, nutritional, environmental, situational and perhaps even emotional predispositions. The bacterium was a necessary but not a sufficient cause in itself for the development of clinically apparent tuberculosis. Today, we have a conception of disease as a form of disordered physiology defined in terms of a concatenation of manifestations which occur together with statistical frequency. This disorder of functioning appears to follow upon the action of a specific etiological agent or agents acting in a setting favourably prepared for disease onset by some characteristics of the prospective patient, as well as by noxious physical, social and psychologic influences from his environment. This definition of disease would encompass all entities ranging from a lacerated scalp due to a blow on the head, to parasitic infestation of the liver in a Chinese peasant. There is another aspect to our modern conception of disease which bears mentioning, and which links with the ancient idea of an equilibrium of forces. Many manifestations of disease are now seen not so much as disturbances of equilibrium, but as a result of the body's attempt to restore equilibrium, or what is often called 'homeostasis', hence they are reactive in nature.

How do mental illnesses fit into this kind of conceptualization of disease? Problems of definition and conceptualization are central to the validity of all studies of social influences upon mental disorder and these will be discussed at some length in the next chapter.

2 The Concept of Mental Illness

Just as paleopathology has shown us that physical disease has always been the unhappy lot of mankind, so ancient texts tell us that there have always been individuals whose behaviour, demeanour, speech and manner have been considered so odd by their tribe, village, city or nation as to merit a separate label of deviance. They could be labelled as being demon-possessed, a witch, a sorcerer or God-intoxicated, or they could have been fitted into the general notion of disease and illness and conceptualized as falling into the category of 'patient'. The opinion that such individuals are mentally ill is also an ancient one. A nosology of mental disorders was already in use in ancient Greece and was utilized by Galen. It must be stated at the outset that today this conception is under frontal attack. Henry B. Adams (1964), an American psychologist, says 'There is no such thing as a mental illness in any significantly meaningful sense. Mental illness is a phenomenon involving interpersonal behaviour, not a health or a medical problem.' Professor Thomas Szasz (1961) maintains that the traditional definition of psychiatry is based on false substantives and that psychiatry is thus similar to pseudo-sciences such as alchemy and astrology. He also regards mental illness as a myth based on faulty definitions. In his book *The Myth of Mental Illness*, he focuses particularly on the phenomenon known as hysteria, which he selected for the following reasons:

Historically, it is the problem that captured the attention of the pioneer neuropsychiatrists (e.g. Charcot, Janet, Freud) and led to the gradual differentiation of neurology and psychiatry.
Logically, hysteria brings into focus the need to distinguish bodily illness from imitations of such illness. It thus presented the

physician with the task of distinguishing the 'real' or genuine from the 'unreal' or false. The distinction between fact and facsimile – often apprehended as the distinction between object and sign, or between physics and psychology – remains the core problem of contemporary psychiatric epistemology.

→ *Psychosocially*, conversion hysteria provides an excellent example of how so-called mental illness can best be conceptualized in terms of sign-using, rule-following and game-playing because: (a) hysteria is a form of nonverbal communication, making use of a special set of signs. (b) It is a system of rule-following behavior, making special use of the rules of helplessness, illness and coercion. (c) It is a game characterized among other things, by the end-goals of domination and interpersonal control and by strategies of deceit. Everything that will be said about hysteria pertains equally, in principal, to all other so-called mental illnesses and to personal conduct generally.

This quotation encapsulates very well Szasz's belief that so-called mental illness is merely a metaphor and moreover a metaphor calculatingly used by certain powerful forces (often malign ones) to stigmatize people as being mentally ill. He believes that these people merely have problems in living, problems which have no basis in disordered physiology. He further asserts that judgements as to 'mental illness' are really based on ethical, social and doctrinaire thinking. His work has been eagerly taken up by a wide variety of individuals who wish to do away with any medical model of mental disease. There are those, professional or otherwise, who wish to call patients 'clients' or 'students' and who wish to treat these clients or students by correcting their supposed difficulties in living, in interpersonal relationships or in learning. It must be said that many psychiatrists regard the nomenclature of these reconstructive efforts, perhaps unfairly, as being in some cases disingenuous. They feel this verbiage clothes attempts on the part of non-medical individuals to take charge of the treatment of humans whom psychiatrists and other physicians would regard as falling into the category of 'patient' and hence appropriately treated only under the direction of a medical practitioner. In practical terms, the controversy generally revolves around the diagnosis and treatment of those individuals whose disturbances of mood, thought or behaviour are relatively mild. Individuals with very severe deviations from the norm in these directions are generally ones whose treatment or 're-education' is left to the medical profession. Although one admires the dextrous and subtle philosophical and epistemological arguments of Szasz, still the fact remains that he has made few medical converts and that his arguments are considered sophistry by many, even though they find it difficult to contradict him on purely intellectual and theoretical grounds. In this connection the arguments of Bishop George Berkeley in the eighteenth century come immediately to mind. Berkeley argued that material objects exist only through the medium of being perceived. Since it is presumed that they are being continuously perceived by God they have a continuous rather than a disconnected existence. A limerick by Ronald Knox quoted by Bertrand Russell (1946) in his *A History of Western Philosophy* is apposite.

There was a young man who said, God
Must think it exceedingly odd
    If he finds that this tree
    Continues to be
When there's no one about in the Quad.

Reply

Dear Sir: Your astonishment's odd:
I am always about in the Quad.
    And that's why the tree
    Will continue to be,
Since observed by yours faithfully, God.

It is said that when Dr Samuel Johnson was informed of the Berkeleian thesis and asked how he would reply to it, he kicked an object and said, 'I refute it thus'. Of course, the kick was no proper refutation of the philosophical argument at all, yet it has a certain persuasive quality about it. Similarly, most people who work in hospitals, clinics or other treatment centres, find it difficult to believe that all the patients whom they are seeing and treating are victims of a linguistic myth and are merely playing some reciprocal game with the authorities of society. The patients do not go away. They are not exorcized by this conceptualization of myth, and the nagging fact of the ubiquity of certain unique combinations of symptoms remains.

Siegler and Osmond (1966) have examined the entire range of theories or models which attempt to classify the serious mental disorder called schizophrenia. Their arguments apply equally well to other major emotional and behavioural disturbances. They have sorted all the theories into six models – medical, moral, psychoanalytic, family interactional, conspiratorial and social. In the medical model, the disorder in the individual is given a definition or a diagnosis. The diagnosis, be it schizophrenia, reactive depression, anxiety reaction or whatever, is considered to be a disorder in the individual's functioning which is mediated through the actual physical nervous system, particularly the brain. The diagnoses of mental illness are considered to be analogous to those in other areas of medicine, for example, diagnoses such as cancer or appendicitis. This diagnostic model implies an etiology or causation exists for each disease. In the case of most mental illnesses it is as yet unknown; however in some, such as delirious intoxications due to various drugs, the psychiatric syndromes associated with brain damage due to syphilis, or more recently the association of depressive mental illness with recognizable changes in the chemical constituents of body fluids, the etiology may be largely or partially discovered. In the medical model the patient's behaviour is interpreted as giving a clue, albeit often an inadequate one, as to the severity of the illness. Treatment consists of procedures of a medical or occasionally of a surgical nature, carried out by appropriately trained medical personnel, that is, by psychiatrists, nurses, attendants, clinically trained psychologists, medical social workers etc. The patient is treated in a hospital, clinic or other medical setting, and will leave the treatment institution when his physician feels that he is well enough to leave without danger to himself or others. The patient and his family have certain rights and duties similar to those of any other patients with serious physical illnesses. Society has the right and the duty to protect its well members from mentally ill persons but is expected to be sympathetic and helpful in creating treatment possibilities for them. This is the medical model of mental disturbance, and it is a model which, at the moment, is clearly predominant although not without challenge.

In the moral model the concern is with the patient's unacceptable behaviour which violates the mores of a given society. There is felt to be no illness, and the behaviour itself is the primary or exclusive concern of those involved with the individual's care. Treatment is carried on in some form of correctional institution, principally hospital, and involves a spectrum of treatments ranging from moral exhortation to various forms of behaviour therapy and conditioning or deconditioning. Practitioners under this model would include individuals such as experimental psychologists or ministers. In this model medical treatment and any form of depth psychotherapy, particularly psychoanalysis, which attempts to understand in psychodynamic terms the patient's manifestations, is to be condemned.

In the psychoanalytic model, which (in its extreme form as regards diagnosis) is strongly advocated by such eminent figures as Dr Karl Menninger (1968), there is felt to be a continuum of emotional difficulties ranging from mild disturbances to severe psychosis. The emotional problems of the most disturbed are felt to be merely quantitatively, rather than qualitatively, different from those of the least disturbed. In this model there is no need for any kind of formal taxonomy or exact classification, and diagnosis is unnecessary. The etiology of the disturbances is thought to relate to unfortunate experiences in early childhood. The patient's behaviour and speech are to be interpreted in terms of their supposed symbolic significance.

In the family interaction model, the whole family is felt to be sick, and the task of the therapist is to conduct group therapy in which all the various intrafamilial manoeuvres, which are alleged to be responsible for the patient's disturbance, are identified, examined, clarified and expunged.

The conspiratorial model is scarcely an inclusive model but

purports to show that individuals who are troublemakers in any group whether the group be the family, the army, the company or the school, are labelled as being 'mentally ill' and are incarcerated in total institutions. The terrible experience of being enveloped in such a hideous, repressive and all-encompassing environment from which they cannot escape is said to account for their subsequent bizarre behaviour. The psychological treatments that the patient undergoes in these institutions are conceived in this model to be purely enforced indoctrination or brainwashing. Therapists are regarded as agents of society attempting to impose a particular point of view on unwilling individuals whom they have incorrectly labelled as ill.

Finally, in the social model, the mental illness is felt to be related to the malfunctioning of the individual's society. The concept of a 'sick' society is one which has a current vogue but, as will be seen presently, there is a good deal of information which casts doubt on the thesis that our present society is responsible for marked increases in serious mental illness.

Obviously, some of these models are grossly incomplete and it may well be that in most institutions today some combination of the models is used in the ratiocinations of the staff without being made explicit in most instances. In any case, the medical model is the most thoroughly worked out of all, and comprehension of its major tenets and of its use is necessary to the understanding of any of the major studies concerning social factors in mental illness. The medical model received much support many decades ago with the demonstration of the association of psychiatric syndromes with clear-cut structural changes in the brain, or with particular disorders of the body's metabolism. However, in none of the major mental illnesses were pathologists able to document causative pathological central nervous system changes. Nevertheless, recent advances in the neurochemistry of the brain have led to the belief that certain abnormalities of the chemical transmitters of neural impulses may be associated with the etiology of the major psychiatric diseases.

Even within the ranks of those who accept the cogency of

the medical model there are many who have raised substantial objections to the current psychiatric taxonomies. The reliability as well as the validity of psychiatric diagnoses have been strongly questioned. For instance, a number of studies have been done over the years involving the independent rating of a patient, or a film or video tape of a patient, by psychiatrists or other mental health workers. Diagnostic agreement has been far from 100 per cent. Depending on the studies, agreement has been reached in 54 per cent of cases, 65 per cent of cases and so forth. However, agreements as to major diagnostic categories have always been well above chance, and if a standardized type examination is used a very high degree of reliability indeed can be achieved, particularly if, as Kreitman (1961) points out, variables relating to the psychiatrists, to the psychiatric examination, to nomenclature, to reporting of the interviews, to the patients, and to the manner of analysis are standardized. That is the psychiatrists doing the rating should be of approximately equal experience, the examinations of a similar type and length, the nomenclature and classification used should be agreed upon in advance, and the patients should be characteristic of those commonly seen by psychiatrists. The type of statistical analysis should also be standardized. The work of Wing (1967) and his co-workers, both at the Maudsley Hospital in London, and abroad, is illuminating in this area.

A technique for the systematic description, measurement and classification of the patient's 'present mental state' by means of a systematic interview, has been developed by Wing. This interview is based upon a checklist of more than 400 items which represent symptoms likely to be encountered in an interview with a patient suffering from one of the functional psychoses or neuroses. The interview to obtain the data necessary for the completion of the schedule is semi-structured and is conducted according to three main principles. First, the examination covers only the patient's present state, from a month before the interview until the present, and not his past history. Second, the schedule is not a questionnaire so that the examiner is at liberty to depart from the order of items during the course of the interview. Thirdly, the schedule is such that each section has a few screening questions which, if answered in the negative, indicate that it is unnecessary for the examiner to proceed to the more detailed protocol. The information obtained is used in the rating of specific symptoms by score: examples of such symptoms would be worrying, anxiety, depression, delusions, hallucinations, etc. Reliability studies were run on 172 patients on whom ratings were made independently by two psychiatrists using the present state interview. On categorization of the patient as to major diagnostic type there was complete agreement in 63 per cent of the cases and partial agreement in 70 per cent, giving an excellent overall concordance rate as compared with previous studies. Similarly, the scores on the individual sections were found to have reliability coefficients as high as 0·95 per cent. This interview schedule is being used in current research and forms the foundation of an interviewing protocol to be used by the World Health Organization in its International Pilot Study of Schizophrenia.

It must not be thought, however, that reliability and standardization of approach are problems confined to psychiatric diagnoses. For example, even in so well defined a disease as leukaemia (cancer of the blood), four research teams from different medical schools were unable to come to an agreement during more than a year of discussions as to the precise definition of a case in a particular form of this disease.

Another difficulty in psychiatric diagnoses is that there are various different bases used in the classification system. For example, in some of the diagnostic categories, such as psychopathic personality, the diagnosis is based upon the individual's antisocial behaviour. The diagnosis of anxiety reaction is made on the evidence of the patient's description of his inner feelings. A third diagnosis, that of chronic brain syndrome associated with arterio-sclerosis, is based partly upon description of and partly upon the demonstration of pathological lesions within the patient's brain and arterial tree. In still another instance, the diagnosis of chronic brain syndrome due to syphilis is based largely upon the etiology of the condition.

Szasz criticized the mixed nature of the classification by stating, 'This is as though in the periodic table of elements we would find coal, steel and petroleum interspersed among items such as helium, sulfur and carbon.'

The designers of the most important classificatory schemes are well aware of this complaint and have attempted to take this objection into account by simultaneously using several axes or bases for classification. In spite of the questionable logic of the use of multiple bases for classification, the method can be surprisingly useful clinically. Various attempts to do away with it thus far have met with limited success. Other general objections to the notion of the classification of mental disorders include the supposed stigma to the patient of having a psychiatric diagnosis and the supposed barrier to progress in psychiatric understanding imposed by a rigid taxonomic system. In the case of the latter objection it is extraordinarily difficult to imagine progress in any science without some taxonomic scheme, however imperfect it might be. It is certainly true that classification has often preceded the discovery of a specific etiology for a disease. For example, general paresis was a recognized clinical entity long before the spirochete of syphilis was demonstrated in the brains of victims. Similarly, pellagrous psychosis was described before the discovery that the disorder was caused by a vitamin deficiency. Phenylketonuria, a syndrome of mental deficiency, was well known before its genetic cause was elucidated.

Increasingly, attempts are made to utilize operational definitions for psychiatric disorders. The concept of the operational definition owes much to the work of the Nobel Laureate physicist, Bridgman (1927), who elucidated the idea in his book *The Logic of Modern Physics*. Hempel (1961) provides a clear exposition of the use of this term:

An operational definition for a given term is conceived as providing objective criteria by means of which any scientific investigator can decide, for any particular case, whether the term does or does not apply to that case. To this end, the operational definition specifies a testing 'operation' T that can be performed on any case to which the given term could conceivably apply, and a certain outcome O of

The Concept of Mental Illness

the testing operation, whose occurrence is to count as the criterion for the applicability of the term to the given case. Schematically, an operational definition of a scientific term S is a stipulation to the effect that S is to apply to all and only those cases for which performance of a test operation T yields the specified outcome O. To illustrate: a simple operational definition of the term *harder than* as used in mineralogy might specify that a piece of mineral x is to be called harder than another piece of mineral y, if the operation of drawing a sharp point of x under pressure across a smooth surface of y has as its outcome a scratch on y, whereas y does not thus scratch x. Similarly, an operational definition of length has to specify rules for the measurement of length in terms of publicly performable operations, such as the appropriate use of measuring rods. Again, phenylpyruvic oligophrenia might be operationally defined by reference to the 'operation' of chemically testing the urine of the person concerned for the presence of phenylpyruvic acid; the 'outcome' indicating the presence of the condition (and thus the applicability of the corresponding term) is simply a positive result of the test. Most diagnostic procedures used in medicine are based on operational criteria of application for corresponding diagnostic categories.

Most psychiatric classification schemes are based on etiological, descriptive or therapeutic response criteria. Many, in fact, use a mixture of all three. To be truly useful, both for purposes of clinical and social psychiatry, a classification should be simple; it should lend itself to being compiled in some orderly statistical fashion; it should attempt to be as universal or all embracing as is possible; and the definitions and terms should be compiled in one manual. Although there are objectionable features to any one of the modern systems of psychiatric classification, the *Diagnostic and Statistical Manual of Mental Disorders* (1968), prepared by the Committee of Nomenclature and Statistics of the American Psychiatric Association, is a most excellent and thorough one. The individuals responsible for its development were psychiatrists, psychologists, statisticians and other scientists who were intimately familiar with all the tribulations and intricacies of psychiatric classification. Materials used in the production of this classification came not merely from the United States but also from the World Health Organization and from experts both in the United Kingdom and on the Continent. The manual has major similarities to the psychiatric sections of the World Health Organization International Classification of Disease (ICD-8). The *Glossary of Mental Disorders* compiled for use in the United Kingdom by the General Register Office also incorporates similar diagnostic categorizations.

There are ten major categories in the diagnostic nomenclature:

1. Mental retardation.

2. Organic brain syndromes. These disorders caused by or associated with impairment of brain tissue function, for example, senile dementia, alcoholic psychosis, psychosis associated with intra-cranial infection, psychosis associated with brain trauma, and so forth.

3. Psychoses not attributed to physical conditions listed previously. This rubric includes schizophrenia, and the so-called major affective disorders including depressions and manias.

4. Neuroses. This includes anxiety neurosis, phobic neurosis, obsessive compulsive neurosis, hypochondrical neurosis, and so forth.

5. Personality disorders, including paranoid personality, psychothymic personalities, schizoid personality, explosive personality, compulsive personality, antisocial personality, etc. Also classified under this category are sexual deviations, alcoholism and drug dependency.

6. Psychophysiological disorders, defined as physical disorders of presumably psychogenic origin involving various body organ systems.

7. Special symptoms not elsewhere classified.

8. Transient situational disturbances.

9. Behaviour disorders of childhood and adolescence.

10. Conditions without manifest psychiatric disorders and non-specific conditions. These conditions include such phenomena as social maladjustments, marital maladjustment, occupational maladjustment and dyssocial behaviour.

The Concept of Mental Illness

The major categories most commonly encountered in social psychiatric studies are those of psychoses without demonstrable etiology, neuroses, personality disorders and psychophysiological (psychosomatic) conditions. The major psychoses described are: first, schizophrenia which is a disorder or a group of disorders manifested by severe and characteristic disturbances of thinking, mood and behaviour. The patient displays illogical and disordering thought and speech patterns and alternations of mood and emotional set including ambivalence, constricted and inappropriate emotional responsiveness, and loss of ordinary emotional give-and-take with others. Behaviour may be withdrawn, peculiar, bizarre or regressive. Delusions and hallucinations may be prominent, particularly in the paranoid type of schizophrenia. Schizophrenia is the disorder which is commonly thought of by laymen when they use the term insanity.

The other major group of psychoses are labelled affective psychoses, and these are characterized by a profound disorder of mood, usually extreme depression or marked and inappropriate elation, which dominates the mental life to the point of unreality. The patient's thinking usually is appropriate to his mood. In the case of the depressed patient, the thoughts are gloomy, full of forebodings, preoccupied with death, destruction, suicide, grief and guilt. The patient's motor activities may be markedly slowed down or extremely agitated or speeded up. In the neuroses the alteration in reality testing, so prominent in the psychoses, is not markedly present. The chief characteristic of the neuroses is anxiety, either expressed directly or controlled unconsciously and automatically by certain mental mechanisms such as conversion or displacement.

The personality disorders are characterized by patterns of behaviour which are maladaptive and life-long. For example, the paranoid personality who is extraordinarily suspicious, envious, jealous, rigid, touchy and liable to sudden rages finds his life seriously impaired by his faulty personality structure. Similarly the schizoid personality who is excessively seclusive, eccentric, shy and grossly withdrawn is also handicapped.

In the psychosomatic disorders, there are characteristically physical symptoms involving various organ systems which appear to result from emotional difficulties. For example, in psychogenic reactions involving the cardiovascular system, the patient might exhibit rapid heartbeat, high blood pressure or migraine headaches. Similarly, in psychophysiological gastrointestinal disorders the patient might show chronic gastritis, excess acidity, constipation, irritable colon and so forth.

To an investigator in the field of mental illness, particularly the psychiatric investigator who accepts this or a similar classification, any individuals coming to his attention to whom one of these diagnostic labels could be applied would be defined as a 'case'. A World Health Organization Expert Committee on Mental Health suggests as an operational definition of a case,

a manifest disturbance of mental functioning specific enough in clinical character to be consistently recognizable as conforming to a clearly defined standard pattern and severe enough to cause loss of working or social capacity or both of a degree which can be specified in terms of absence from work or the taking of legal or other social action.

Although in this difficult field, a 'press on regardless' attitude may result in disorderly or simple-minded work of limited value, nevertheless, as the late Major Greenwood (1948), one of the great epidemiologists of our day, pointed out: 'Making the best the enemy of the good is a sure way to hinder any statistical progress. The scientific purist, who will wait for medical statistics until they are nosologically exact, is no wiser than Horace's rustic waiting for the river to flow away.'

3 The Epidemiology of Mental Illness

If one were interested in the problem of how common a disease is and what sort of people it most affects, one would think immediately of examining the records of hospitals and physicians. Many mental hospitals are institutions of some antiquity which have kept records of varying quality since they opened their doors. Even in the last century pioneers such as Esquirol in France, Maudsley and Tuke in England, and Earle in America, examined hospital statistics relating to the prevalence of insanity. In all cases they were able to show that there were, in fact, more hospitalized mentally ill patients later in the nineteenth century than there were at the beginning. They wisely, however, did not attribute this apparent increase to an actual increase in overall prevalence of mental illness in the community but rather they speculated that there had been certain environmental changes which had brought about the increase in hospitalized patients.

First and foremost, the availability of beds in hospital for the mentally ill is paramount in the determination of the number of people hospitalized. Similarly, *mutatis mutandis*, the availability of out-patient facilities often determines the number of ambulatory patients recorded. Most communities then and now, at least until the onset of the era of psychotropic drugs, have not had anything like a sufficiency of beds in hospital, so that many prospective patients were not hospitalized in spite of need. Other factors implicit in the decision to hospitalize include the cost of hospitalization and the ready availability of alternative health resources within the community, for example, private psychiatrists, community clinics, psychiatric facilities in general hospitals and university clinics. There are, of course, many more alternative treatment facilities available at present than in the past, not only community clinics but also chronic disease hospitals, nursing homes, old people's homes, and so forth.

Another factor of enormous importance in the rate of hospital admissions is the legal code relating to insanity and commitment. For example, in England, in the last century, following the passage of the Lunacy Acts which facilitated hospital admission for the mentally ill, the number of admissions rose very steeply indeed. Similarly, hospital admissions are also strongly influenced by community feelings about mental illness and its care. For example, if in a given culture certain kinds of aberrant behaviour are not conceived of as representing mental illness, then, of course, no treatment will be sought for those possessing these manifestations. Similarly, if it is the community feeling that disturbances of mood or behaviour are best treated at home and that hospitals are institutions to be avoided except in dire extremity, then clearly admission rates will be far from reflecting the true incidence or prevalence of mental disorder within the community. What is true for the community is *a fortiori* true for the medical profession. Obviously, in any society the medical profession is the major channel through which cases flow into mental hospitals. The physician's concept of what constitutes mental illness and its correct care will clearly influence whether or not he will admit a patient to hospital. Also the decision of the patient, his family, the physician, or in some cases the courts, will be influenced by the location of hospitals in relation to the community.

Another item influencing the decision for hospitalization is the kind of reputation that the hospitals possess. For example, both in the past and to a lesser extent today, large public hospitals (called state hospitals in America) have had a rather unfavourable reputation and there was great hesitation in sending a patient to such an institution because the act of commitment was equated in the public mind with forcing the individual into a vile and inescapable situation.

Thus the total hospitalized population in a given geographical area at a given point in time, that is, the point prevalence of hospitalized psychiatric patients, is a reflection not only of the true prevalence of mental disorders but also of a wide variety of social factors which influence the decision for admission.

The hospital prevalence figures also depend upon the patient's length of stay within the mental hospital. In turn, the length of stay of any given patient with a mental disease in hospital depends, in part, upon the severity and course of his illness. Nevertheless, the clinical picture is by no means the only nor perhaps even the major criterion utilized by the hospital staff in gauging the appropriate length of stay for the patient. It was shown by Bockoven (1963) and others, that in the first half of the nineteenth century, both in England and in America, mental patients had relatively short stays in hospital where they were treated by what was then known as 'moral treatment' which was essentially a form of milieu therapy combined with hortatory advice. It was expected that the patients would get better under this kindly regimen and early discharge was commonplace. As the century wore on, particularly in America, massive increases in population, primarily by immigration, flooded the hospitals with more patients than they could reasonably handle. Moreover, the patients were often of a different ethnic background and social class from the patients seen some decades before; there was less in common between patients and physicians and hence little rapport between them. Simultaneously, the idea of organic causation of all illnesses, including mental ones, was beginning to triumph. An extremely pessimistic view of prognosis in mental illness developed and it was felt that most patients would need to be hospitalized for the rest of their lives. This proved to be a self-fulfilling prophecy and by the turn of the century the mental hospitals were crowded almost beyond belief with individuals who were fated to remain there for decades. This bleak outlook has been drastically changed over the past fifteen years and now once again there is general expectation that most people who are admitted to a mental hospital will sooner or later, more often sooner, be returned to the community. There is a pervasive feeling of therapeutic optimism at present which facilitates the early discharge of hospitalized patients, and consequently, standards relating to discharge have changed and individuals are returned to society still exhibiting many symptoms. Heretofore, hospital staff would have felt remissed in their duties, both toward the patient and society, if they had released patients in such condition, but today they feel otherwise. They assert that early discharge, even though the patient may still have some symptoms, prevents the development of the regressive behaviour fostered by the hospital setting and that the patient will do better being treated in an out-patient rather than an in-patient setting. With the introduction of chlorpromazine for general use in 1954, potent drugs became available for the first time in psychiatric practice. Some of these could control agitation and psychotic turmoil and others appeared to be associated with alleviation of depressive illnesses. These drugs and the therapeutic enthusiasm they provoked also served to shorten the duration of stay in the mental hospital.

Still other factors which determine the size of the total inpatient population include the type and seriousness of illness, the death rates among in-patients, and their age range. For example, mental hospitals in some countries have very high death rates from such concurrent or intercurrent physical illnesses as tuberculosis or dysentery. A hospital with a large percentage of geriatric patients will, of course, have a high death rate. It would appear at present that we are in an era where first admission and readmission rates continue to climb but where the duration of patient stay is short (particularly for the younger age group) and where the vast bulk of patients can expect to be discharged (see Figure 1). In the New Hampshire (USA) mental hospital population at present, Bryce *et al.* (1966) report that 50 per cent of all admissions are readmissions and 50 per cent of all readmissions are multiple readmissions, that is patients who have had two or more previous admissions. In California, the rate of readmissions to state mental hospitals for the period 1962 to 1967 exceeded the rate of first admissions by more than nineteen to one. In spite of a high readmission rate the resident mental hospital population of a large state like New York has been dropping at the rate of

1 to 1·5 per cent per annum which is about the overall national rate. The figures in the United Kingdom reflect the same general trends.

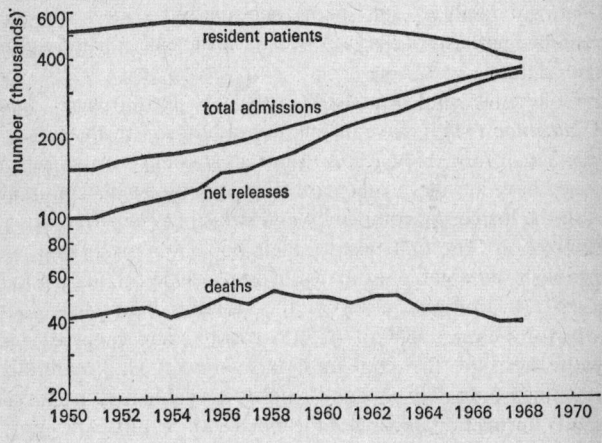

Figure 1 Number of resident patients, total admissions, net releases and deaths, state and county mental hospitals, United States, 1950–68
Source: *Mental Health Statistics*, Current Facility Reports, US Department of Health, Education and Welfare, Public Health Service, National Institute of Mental Health.

In a study of a recent series of schizophrenic patients in a naval hospital, it was found that over 95 per cent of these patients were returned either to civil life or to duty within a year, and that only one out of twenty required long-term hospitalization in an old people's hospital. This is in marked contrast to the experience of even twenty years before where 30 to 40 per cent of such patients would have been expected to remain in hospital for more than a year.

In spite of the methodological problems associated with the research use of hospitalization rates, many intensive studies have been carried out which utilize such data in an attempt to ascertain the incidence and prevalence of mental illness of a serious nature in different population groups. Hospitalization rates have been used by scientists to make inferences about a number of social, environmental, economic, cultural and other variables involved in the prevalence of mental illness. Data of this kind have been used by administrators in planning treatment facilities, and many speculations concerning the changing patterns of disease occurrence have been based upon such data.

Goldhamer and Marshall, in their book *Psychosis and Civilization* (1949), have ingeniously addressed themselves to the task of furnishing at least a partial answer to the question concerning an alleged increase in mental illness concomitant with the increasing complexity and stress of twentieth century civilization. The first task of their book was an attempt to establish 'acceptable estimates of age-specific first-admission rates to institutions caring for the mentally ill in Massachusetts for the years 1840 to 1855 in order to compare these rates with those of the contemporary period'. They carefully examined the relatively good records available relating to insanity during that portion of the nineteenth century. They were able to enumerate those cases which, although the diagnostic naming has since changed, seemed to represent clearcut psychosis as we would judge it today. When they compared similar types of patients of similar age they found that age-specific first-admission rates for individuals under fifty were just as high in the nineteenth century as they are today. On the other hand, there was a very marked increase in admission rates in the old age group in the modern era. This appeared to be primarily due to an increase in the facilities available for the care of such patients and to changing social conditions which facilitated the hospitalization of those older people who, in Victorian times would have remained within the bosom of their families. In addition there may well have been an increase in patients with arterio-sclerotic brain disease. They concluded, 'there has been no long-term increase during the last century in the incidence of the psychoses of early and middle life'. Their work applies particularly to the functional psychoses such as schizophrenia. The study of long-term rather than short-term trends did not discuss at all the problems of minor mental illness of the psychoneurotic or personality disorder variety.

Further corroboration of the stable character of hospital admission rates for functional psychoses is provided by the work of Arthur (1965), who examined the rates of insanity in the United States Navy over the past sixty years. He was able to show that the psychosis admission rate had remained remarkably constant in spite of the changing size and composition of the Navy during two World Wars and numerous other momentous events. The rate has always been approximately one to one and a half admissions per thousand Navy men on active duty per annum. This figure was thought to be reasonably close to the true incidence rate of severe psychosis since the number of beds in the naval hospitals are theoretically unlimited in that any Navy man who is designated by a medical officer for admission to a naval hospital must be admitted. Furthermore, the close scrutiny and crowded living conditions implicit in naval life make it unlikely that anyone whose speech, mood or behaviour is markedly aberrant could escape official notice. This stability of rate applied only to psychotic disorders such as schizophrenia. The rates of admission to naval hospitals for psychoneuroses and personality disorders fluctuated very markedly depending on the overall situation. For example, the rates for these latter disorders went up sharply during the Second World War and the Korean War and dropped equally sharply after the cessation of hostilities.

Morton Kramer (1969), Chief of the Biometrics Branch of the US National Institute of Mental Health, has written extensively on the topic of hospitalization rates for mental disorders. His study of US national statistics has shown declining admission rates for psychoses associated with syphilis. This seems to be a genuine indicator of the diminishing importance of this disease. His data have also shown a decrease in the admission rate of manic-depressive psychosis. This fact has been interpreted in many ways with opinion divided as to whether this reduction is due to artefacts relating to changing fashions in psychiatric diagnosis or whether there has been a genuine decrease in the incidence and prevalence of this disorder. Kramer also studied first-admission rates to mental hospitals in the US as compared to those of the mental hospitals of England and Wales. The rates were specific for sex, age and diagnosis. He was able to document several important points: first, the total admission rates for all disorders was virtually the same for both nations, that is, the age-adjusted rate per 100,000 population per annum was 102·1 in the US and 115·7 in England and Wales in 1960. However, the diagnostic categories into which the patients were fitted were rather different. The first-admission rate for schizophrenia was about one-third lower in England and Wales than in the United States. Similarly, the rate of admissions for psychoses associated with cerebral arterio-sclerosis in the US was ten times that of England and Wales whereas the first-admission rate for manic-depressive psychosis in England and Wales was nine times that of the US. A considerable amount of research has been going on to explain these differences in admission rates and the results of some of this research will be commented on at greater length in chapter 6. Kramer feels that in spite of all the difficulties attendant upon the use of mental hospital statistics, these data have proved very useful for such purposes as

suggesting various hypotheses concerning the distribution of mental disorders, for delineating population groups in which high rates of disability exist, for estimating probabilities of eventually being admitted to mental hospitals, for determining the cost of care of specific groups of patients, and for clarifying analyses of changes in hospital release and death rates.

Pugh and MacMahon (1962), in their work *Epidemiologic Findings in United States Mental Hospital Data* in which they analysed information obtained from all the areas of the United States, showed an increase of first admissions to mental hospitals during the first half of the century for all ages and both sexes. However, they confirmed that there had been very little long-term change in admission rates for the psychotic disorders category. The increases had come primarily in other types of mental illness such as psychoneuroses and personality disorders. The data also showed that there were high prevalence rates of hospitalization for mental illness in the foreign-born than in the native-born; higher rates among the non-white than in the white; and higher rates for the single, widowed, separated or divorced persons than for the married. There was a short-term increase in admission rates for mental disorders in young males in the USA during the Second World War in contrast to the experience in several European countries where a decrease in admissions occurred. The order of magnitude of the admission rates in males for psychotic disorders in 1945 approximated 46·1 first admissions per 100,000 population at risk. For females the corresponding figure was 46·8 admissions per 100,000 persons at risk for the year.

Vera Norris (1959), in her book *Mental Illness in London*, utilized information derived from mental hospitals which showed psychosis admission rates for London to be higher than those for an essentially rural county such as Buckinghamshire but to be somewhat lower than those of the United States as a whole and much lower than those of New York. Even in England and Wales, Norris indicated that 'the probability that any individual requires to be admitted at least once to a mental hospital during his life-time is alarmingly high: of the order of 5 per cent; that is to say, one out of every twenty babies born is likely to require hospital treatment for a mental disorder.' This statement was based on admission data for the years 1947–9. There is no reason to believe that the risk has lessened: in fact, it may be greater at present. Shepherd (1957), in his book *A Study of the Major Psychoses in an English County* (Buckinghamshire), also offers a lucid analysis and demonstration of the intelligent use of hospital statistics to delineate the extent of the problem of mental illness in a specified geographical region.

Finally, Gunderson, Arthur and Richardson (1968) utilized hospitalization data in the Navy to clarify relationships between military status and psychiatric admission rates. They showed that the admission rate for unrated enlisted men was more than twice of that for petty officers, and that for petty officers was more than twice that for officers. This was particularly true for the diagnostic categories of psychoneurosis and personality disorders. Psychotic admission rates were relatively constant in the various ranks except for a markedly higher rate amongst the young unrated enlisted men.

The Scandinavian countries have long been models of efficiency in the development of health and illness information on their populations. Statistics relating to mental illness have been gathered there for more than a century. The populations of the countries are quite homogeneous and relatively stable so that relatively complete demographic information is easier possible to obtain than in large nations with considerable immigration and with a heterogeneous population. Ødegård (1968) has made careful studies of hospitalization in Norway and feels that it is possible to make some extrapolations from hospital admission data to figures of actual incidence and prevalence within the community. His data have shown a relative stability of admission rates from 1926 to 1956 excepting only the war years during the German occupation. Since 1956, Norway, in common with the other nations, has shown a decline in the number of patients actually in hospital at any given time in spite of an increase in the readmission rate.

In order to substitute for or to complement available hospital statistics certain investigators have employed data obtained from private practice, either of a psychiatric or general nature, in an attempt to assess the amount of mental illness prevalent in a community. Jaco (1959) carried out a survey of the incidence of psychotic disorders in the entire state of Texas for a two-year period, 1951–2. He surveyed all inhabitants of Texas who sought psychiatric treatment for an illness that was subsequently diagnosed as psychosis for the first time during this period. He obtained his data from private, state, city, county and old people's administration hospitals in Texas and surrounding states, as well as information from every psychiatrist in private practice in Texas during the period in question. He compiled an annual rate which was computed not only for the state as a whole but for various subregions of that state. The incidence rates were adjusted for age, sex and major ethnic compositions of each of the subregions. Standardization of the rates was made by using data from the 1950 census of Texas for population at risk figures, supplemented by a special census. During this period 11,298 individuals were diagnosed for the first time as having a psychosis. The actual figures are shown in Table 3. He further examined the incidence rate not only in terms of sex and ethnic differences but also of occupation, marital status and education.

Table 3 Annual-Adjusted Incidence Rates of Psychoses by Diagnosis of Mexican, Anglo-American and Non-White Groups of Texas, 1951–2, per 100,000 Population

	Males			Females		
	Mexican	Anglo-Americans	Non-white	Mexican	Anglo-Americans	Non-white
Functional	24	47	32	35	69	35
schizophrenia	20	32	30	26	43	32
affective	3	11	2	7	19	2
involutional	1	4	1	2	7	1
Old-age	7	13	11	5	10	10
cerebral arteriosclerosis	4	7	6	2	5	4
senile dementia	3	6	3	3	4	4
Organic	8	13	15	3	7	4
toxic	2	6	4	0	2	1
paresis	4	2	8	1	1	3
other	2	5	4	2	4	1

Source: Jaco (1959, ch. 21, p. 474)

His principal findings were that:

1. The incidence rate of psychoses for Mexican residents in Texas was less than that of the Anglo-American or other groups in the State.

2. Incidence rates for psychoses tended to increase with age.

3. Urban rates were higher than rural rates.

4. There were occupational differences in incidence rates.

As is the case in virtually every study, incidence rates adjusted for age, sex and ethnic differentials were highest for the divorced, followed in order by the single, separated, the widowed and finally the married.

It has long been apparent that data obtained from hospital records, even if supplemented by information from private practitioners, will at best only approximate to true incidence rates. There are obviously individuals who are mentally ill who have not yet come to the attention of the medical profession and hence are not yet counted as a 'case'. Thus, there is a latent period between the onset of symptoms and the labelling of an individual as a case. In an attempt to obviate this and other barriers to the development of true incidence rates, field surveys have been initiated. These surveys include household interviews, large-scale brief psychiatric examinations and the development of first-hand demographic community and social information.

As far back as 1916 Rosanoff (1916) conducted a community survey of mental illness in Nassau County, New York, and arrived at a prevalence figure of 36·4 per thousand population. Since that time there have been innumerable such studies, for example, studies by Cohen, Fairbank and Greene (1938a, b; 1939a, b), and by Lemkau, Tietze and Cooper (1943a, b, c, d) in the Eastern Health District of Maryland, studies by Eaton and Weil (1955) in Hutterite communities in America, and Lin (1966) in Formosa. The value of the studies for comparative purposes has been weakened by their enormous variability of scope, the differing case criteria used, the utilization of differing taxonomic instruments, and even the lack of uniform classification of demographic information, particularly relating to such items as social class. In addition, widely different methods were employed, for example, personal interviews by psychiatrists, personal interviews by other health professionals, interviews by students or trained laymen, structured interviews, semi-structured interviews, free interviews, questionnaires, etc. The data were analysed in many different ways. Ratings of inter-observer reliability were obtained in some studies, not in others. The use of idiosyncratic statistical approaches occurred in some. In others there were ambiguous uses of the terms incidence and prevalence and in the mathematical handling of the differing populations at risk. In spite of these defects the field studies are of crucial importance to the understanding of social psychiatry. Several important examples of field surveys of defined districts seeking the incidence or prevalence of mental illness in a particular social setting will be presented.

A landmark study both in terms of magnitude and impact is the 'Midtown Manhattan' study of Srole, Langner, Michael, Opler and Rennie (1962). The primary objective of the study was to test the very general hypothesis that 'biosocial and sociocultural factors leave imprints on mental health which are discernible when viewed from the panoramic perspective provided by large populations'. In order to obtain information germane to the major thesis of the study, it was first necessary to attempt to ascertain the overall occurrence of mental illness, both treated and untreated, within the defined district. The Midtown district on the East Side of Manhattan was one of 400 city blocks with the very high population density of 140,000 people per square mile. Within the district dwelt approximately 174,000 individuals (99 per cent white) of whom 110,000 were aged twenty to fifty-nine. There was a broad range of socio-economic status represented in the area. The investigators used three approaches to data gathering: the 'Community Sociographic Operation' which was an attempt to elucidate the major sociographic characteristics of the environment particularly those of institutions such as the family, the schools, the police, religious, political and economic structures, and so forth; the 'Treatment Census Operation' which established a point prevalence of all treated psychiatric cases who were residents of the area on 1 May 1953 (some 2240 in all) and who were patients of any of four types of psychiatric facilities – public mental hospitals, private mental hospitals, out-patient clinics and the offices of private practitioners; and the 'Sample Survey Operation' or 'Home Interview Survey' which involved a long questionnaire interview of a random sample of 1911 individuals selected to be representative of the universe of

174,000 inhabitants, of whom 13 per cent of the 1911 did not participate in the survey so that 1660 were actually interviewed, all previously unknown to the interviewers. There were some 400 questions in the interview schedule including information relating to physical health, mental health, childhood, child–parent relationships, work history, interpersonal relationships and socio-economic factors. These respondents were asked over 100 questions of a psychiatric nature. The psychiatric portion of the questionnaire was primarily derived from the Cornell Medical Index, the Army Neuropsychiatric Screening Adjunct and the Minnesota Multiphase Personality Inventory. The questionnaire was administered by trained professional interviewers who were graduate students or psychiatric social workers. Two psychiatrists independently rated each respondent on the basis of the questionnaire on a seven-point scale ranging from zero – no evidence of symptom formation, symptom free; to six – seriously incapacitated, unable to function. The independent ratings of each psychiatrist were then combined to make a twelve-point total score and 'collapsed' to form four gradations of mental health by making mental health ratings: 0–1, well; 2–3, mild symptoms; 4–5, moderate symptoms; and 6–12, impaired (6–7 marked, 8–9 severe, 10–12 incapacitated). On the basis of psychiatrists' ratings the population in Midtown Manhattan was sorted into the following four psychiatric rating categories in terms of the degree of impairment due to mental or emotional difficulties: 23·4 per cent impaired (either incapacitated or with marked or severe symptoms), 21·8 per cent moderately disturbed, 36·3 per cent mildly disturbed, and 18·5 per cent well. In addition to the determination of the prevalence of psychiatric impairment, the study also established a differential prevalence of types of emotional disorders within the various social classes measured by the respondent's education, occupation, income and rent. The data indicated that severe impairment, particularly of a psychotic type, was more common amongst the lower socioeconomic status respondents. The upper classes were found to be receiving psychiatric treatment at a higher rate than those in the lower classes. There was a significant relationship of a reverse type between psychiatric symptoms and socio-economic status, that is, the lower the class the higher the symptom level. This was true even if one considered only the status of a respondent's parents rather than his own – if one had parents in the high status group, one tended to have a low level of symptoms. The downwardly mobile were found to have a significant amount of impairment, more than either the stationary or the upwardly mobile.

Another major study which also involved an interdisciplinary team approach using psychiatrists, psychologists, sociologists and other professionals, is the Stirling County Study of Leighton (1961) and others. The area studied was a rural county in the Canadian province of Nova Scotia and the study attempted to explore how psychiatric disorders and the social and cultural aspects of a given environment might be related. The investigators hoped to discover the effects of certain socio-cultural factors on the origin, course, and prognosis of psychiatric diseases. In addition they wished to compare the distribution of disorders with certain aspects of the environment in a way that might be useful for future planning of treatment and preventive facilities. The investigation began with a prevalence study in an attempt to gain an exact measure of the prevalence of psychiatric disorders amongst the non-hospitalized adult population of Stirling County. Psychiatric disorder was defined in terms of the descriptions used in the *Diagnostic and Statistical Manual of Mental Disorders*, second edition, of the American Psychiatric Association. The investigators also attempted to work out an operational definition of the socio-cultural environment, a task potentially even more difficult than that of delineating psychiatric disorders. Nevertheless, the investigators projected ten major indices used to rate a community as to whether it was 'integrated' or 'disintegrated' in terms of the stability of its environment. The ten indices were as follows:

1. Poverty – instability of income as well as low level.
2. Cultural confusion – that is to say, weak, confused and conflicting values (French and English).
3. Secularization, or in other words, the absence of religious values.

4. Frequency of broken homes.
5. Few and weak associations in the group, both formal and informal.
6. Few and weak leaders.
7. Few patterns of recreation and leisure time activity.
8. High frequency of hostile acts and expressions.
9. High frequency of crime and delinquency.
10. Weak and fragmented network of communications.

The basic hypothesis being tested stated that 'social disintegration generates disintegrated personalities'. The investigators attempted, through field work, to see if communities could be rated as to their functional integrity. Communities identified as being high on the ten indices of sociocultural disintegration were hypothesized to be ones which fostered the development of emotional difficulties in their inhabitants.

The total population of the county was approximately 20,000, divided almost equally between French-Canadians and English-speaking peoples of Scots, Irish or English derivation. The largest town in the county had a population of approximately 3000. Fishing, farming and lumbering were the major occupations. A sample of 1015 persons over the age of eighteen (essentially equally divided between males and females) thought to be representative of the entire universe of the adults in the county was selected. Each person in the sample was interviewed according to a standard questionnaire. In addition, the interviewers assessed the respondent and his household. The ten physicians in general practice in the area were also, within the framework of medical ethics, questioned about the respondent's current health status and past health history as well as about their emotional and social functioning. The records of two general hospitals and four metropolitan hospitals in the main city of the province were also examined. Initially, data concerning each respondent were rated separately by four psychiatrists who then pooled their separate ratings into a mutually agreed final judgement. Later the number of psychiatrist judges was reduced to two. The material was presented to the psychiatrists without the patient's name being apparent nor was there any indication as to whether the patient came from the French-speaking or English-speaking community. The respondents were rated as to the probability and degree of symptoms and impairment. Symptom complexes were evaluated in terms of diagnostic category and as to whether they were current or past. Opinions as to the duration of the symptom patterns and the degree to which the person was impaired, particularly in terms of work, were made by the psychiatrists.

At least half of the adults in Stirling County were thought to be currently suffering from some defined psychiatric disorder, mostly of a mild type, but about one-quarter or more of the population had suffered significant impairment from psychiatric disorder at some point during their lives. A rating was made with regard to the probability that the individual had a psychiatric disorder ranging from 'A' – those almost certainly psychiatrically disordered to 'D' – those virtually free of symptoms. In addition, a rating of degree of impairment was separately made. There was a later modification of the rating of need for psychiatric attention. However, in terms of the A, B, C, D rating, 30·5 per cent belonged in the A category, that is, almost certainly psychiatric cases; the B or probably a psychiatric case category embraced 24·6 per cent of the population; the C or possibly a psychiatric case group 26·2 per cent, and the D or asymptomatic group 18·7 per cent of the total county sample of heads of household eighteen years old or over – findings not dissimilar to the prevalences of emotional impairment found in the city dwellers interviewed in Midtown Manhattan.

The Stirling County investigators felt that the prevalence of psychoses was approximately of the degree expected, that is, rather low. They were surprised, however, at the high prevalence of personality, psychophysiological and psychoneurotic disorders, particularly the latter. However, although the prevalence of significant symptoms was great, the degree of impairment in most individuals was felt not to be vast. Apparently a very large number of people who were getting along relatively well in terms of the ordinary demands of occupational life were nevertheless unhappy and troubled by their symptoms, or a source of difficulty to others, or both. The study also showed that women had a higher prevalence of psychiatric disorder than did men. However, the impairment levels in both sexes were much the same. Women tended to show more psychophysiological and psychoneurotic patterns than did men and fewer personality disorders of a sociopathic nature. However, in one village, the 'well integrated French-Acadian community' of Lavallée, with a population of about 300, the prevalence rate of psychiatric disorders, particularly amongst the women, was much lower than in the county at large and much lower than amongst the women of Fairhaven in particular, an English-speaking community in the county chosen for comparison in that it was of similar size but in which there was less of a completely supportive social network than in Lavallée. In the so-called disintegrated areas of the county, as gauged by communities with high scores on the ten indices of disintegration, the prevalence rate of psychiatric disorders was high for both sexes. Between the ages of twenty to seventy, the older the person the greater the chance he had to display a psychiatric disorder of significant magnitude. In men there was a levelling off of this tendency from forty until sixty. After seventy, both men and women showed a reduction of prevalence of psychiatric disorder which the investigators argued was real rather than artefactual. They suggested a 'general decrease in striving' and the ability to overlook difficulties as well as a general disengagement from life's daily concerns as the factors responsible for this phenomenon. Finally, the investigators addressed themselves to the question as to why there should be an association between social disintegration and the prevalence of psychiatric disorders. They advanced nine hypotheses which might account for this putative association.

Hypothesis 1: Sociocultural disintegration fosters psychiatric disorder by interfering with physical security, e.g. needs for adequate food, shelter, clothing, sleep and care of physical ailments.
Hypothesis 2: Sociocultural disintegration fosters mental health by the degree to which it permits freedom of sexual expression.
Hypothesis 3: Sociocultural disintegration fosters mental health by

the degree to which it permits freedom of hostile and aggressive expressions.

Hypothesis 4: Sociocultural disintegration fosters psychiatric disorder due to limitations put on the giving and receiving of love.

Hypothesis 5: Social disintegration fosters psychiatric disorder by interfering with the achievement of socially valued ends by legitimate means.

Hypothesis 6: Sociocultural disintegration fosters psychiatric disorder by interfering with spontaneity.

Hypothesis 7: Social disintegration fosters psychiatric disorder by interfering with a person's orientation regarding his place in society.

Hypothesis 8: Social disintegration fosters psychiatric disorder by interfering with a person's sense of membership in a definite human group.

Hypothesis 9: Social disintegration fosters psychiatric disorder by interfering with the individual's sense of membership in a moral order.

The group regarded the first three hypotheses as unlikely and certainly not substantiated by their studies. Hypothesis 4, however, received some support from the interview material as did hypothesis 5. Of hypothesis 6, it was noted that in the disintegrated communities there was more activity of a questionable character that individuals could do and 'get away with' than in the integrated communities. This activity involved mainly areas of sex, aggression and alcoholic consumption which might have negative effects on mental health. Moreover, apathy was a major feature of the overall emotional climate in these villages. The integrated communities provided more helpful, creative and important tasks than did the disintegrated communities. Hypotheses 7 and 8 were felt to be important aspects of group influence on optimum mental and emotional functioning. A sense of 'psychological anomie' or alienation was thought by the social scientists to be characteristic of the inhabitants of depressed areas and to affect their mental health adversely. Furthermore, the disintegrated areas in a county were characterized by cultural confusion and widespread secularization which blighted the individual's sense of membership in a moral order. The results of the study were felt to suggest that those aspects of sociocultural disintegration which appeared to have the most effect on the prevalence of psychiatric symptoms were those which interfered with recognition, love, spontaneity and the sense of being part of a moral order and feeling comfortably right in what one does.

It is probably not unjust to say that these hypotheses would scarcely be said to have been proven in the rigorous sense that proof is usually understood in science. On the other hand, certainly concomitant variation was shown between prevalence rates and 'disintegration' as judged by the indices used. Regardless of one's views on the question of whether the hypotheses regarding the etiological role in mental illness origin of environmental factors of a social and cultural kind were proved by these investigations, the Midtown Manhattan and the Stirling County studies, both of which were products of the famous Cornell Program in Social Psychiatry of the Cornell University School of Medicine in New York City, are landmarks of social psychiatric investigation.

Before leaving the topic of general epidemiological surveys in psychiatry there must be mentioned the psychiatric register approach. In the United States, the National Institute of Mental Health, in cooperation with local authorities, has set up psychiatric registers in such areas as Rochester, New York and the State of Maryland. In the United Kingdom a similar cumulative disease register has been set up by the Social Psychiatric Research Unit directed by Dr J. K. Wing (1966a, b; 1967), at the Maudsley Hospital, London, with the support of the Ministry of Health, to act as a sampling framework against which to compare specific patient populations. This register provides demographic, social and clinical data about all Camberwell residents who contact psychiatric services.

The former LCC Borough of Camberwell is now part of the GLC Borough of Southwark. The psychiatric services of the area are provided by the Cane Hill, Maudsley and King's College Hospitals. Data are collected about all patients receiving any psychiatric service from this geographical area, so that selection bias is avoided. The data from many different agencies, including local authority services, in-patient service, day hospitals, out-patient clinics, emergency clinics, local practitioners and private psychiatrists are collated.

The register began with a census of all Camberwell residents who were in contact with psychiatric services on 31 December 1964, and all contacts since then have been reported. The register is cumulative so that the progress of patients can be followed through time as they move from one agency to another or as new services are introduced. These data provide, (a) unduplicated counts of patients who contact many agencies, (b) a defined population base, and (c) cumulative data, because every patient contact with any agency in the district is to be reported and registered in the patient's dossier. There are approximately 175,000 inhabitants of Camberwell. It is thought that the register is picking up at least 95 per cent of all the psychiatric cases in the district as defined in terms of contact with a psychiatrist. A very few people, indeed, go to Harley Street for private care, and these very affluent patients would be essentially the only source of loss to the register. The register has already been used as a starting point for further studies, for example, a study of schizophrenia in Camberwell.

In this study all the schizophrenic patients who are residents of Camberwell and who are on the register are being studied by means of the present status interviewing and family study techniques previously described. In addition, a period prevalence study is being made in the districts, in which various sub-districts are being sampled by field survey methods with a view to establishing the prevalence of all diagnosable mental disorders, not merely counting those patients who had actually seen a psychiatrist and had had a psychiatric diagnosis made previously. Results thus far indicate that about 2 per cent of the population is on the register as a diagnosed psychiatric case but that approximately 15 per cent of the general sample has a diagnosable psychiatric disorder of varying severity. Further research is projected to answer the question as to why the 13 per cent of Camberwell residents who have a diagnosable psychiatric disorder do not seek psychiatric help as contrasted to the 2 per cent who do.

The register is also being used to collect information about Camberwell residents receiving psychotherapy from any agency within the National Health Service. It will thus be possible to calculate an incidence and prevalence rate for patients receiving psychotherapy.

The register can be used as a starting point for all sorts of important operational studies of psychiatric services. A carefully defined district with well-delineated material on the medical and psychiatric aspects of the population provides an excellent social laboratory.

We might best begin a summary of this chapter by examining Table 4, which is taken from a book by Plunkett and Gordon entitled *Epidemiology and Mental Illness* (1960). The authors' comment on this Table is: 'The range of rates is so great as to defy generalization. Obviously the recorded values are affected strongly by differences in study design, by study definitions and by classification systems.' This appears to be too nihilistic a judgement about the results of those and other studies. It would appear that a distillate of all available studies does disclose some valid generalizations. The first is that the incidence rate of psychotic illness is relatively low in any carefully defined population. However, since the disorders tend to be extremely chronic in nature and have, in the past, involved long periods of hospitalization, the overall prevalence is relatively high because of the accumulation of cases in hospital. The rates of hospitalization for psychotic illness in persons below sixty have tended to be relatively stationary over the long term and to be approximately the same for both sexes, with the highest rates occurring in young men between the ages of twenty and thirty and for women between the ages of forty and fifty. The rates have consistently shown an excess of hospitalization for the single, widowed, separated, divorced and recent immigrant categories.

Field surveys have established a very high prevalence of mild to moderate psychiatric symptoms and various emotional impairments of living in the populations studied. About a

third of the selected populations in locations as dissimilar as
Nova Scotia and New York City were thought by psychiatrists

Table 4 Eleven Community Surveys of Mental Illness
Prevalence Rates per 1000 Population

Survey	Total mental disorders	Psychoses	Neuroses
Nassau County	36·4[a]		
Eastern Health District (1933)	44·5[b]	8·18[b] (over 15)	2·0[b]
Eastern Health District (1936)	60·5[b]	6·6[b] (over 10)	10·7[b]
Tennessee	46·7*[a]	4·9*[a]	3·6*[a]
Hutterite Communities	16·7*[c]	4·7*[c] (15 and over)	11·5*[c] (15 and over)
New Jersey	138·0[a]	2·0[a]	
Baltimore	108·6[a]	4·3[a] (over 16)	52·6[a]
Salt Lake City	circa 333·0[a] (over 16)		
Syracuse (Bellin and Hardt)	232·0[a] (65 and over)		
Syracuse (Downing and Gruenberg)	53·0[a] (65 and over)		
Midtown	233·0[a] ('impaired') (20 to 59)		

* Our calculation
a One-day rate (day of examination or interview considered equivalent to a single day)
b One-year rate
c Three-month rate
Source: Plunkett and Gordon (1960, p. 90)

to have a significant number of psychiatric symptoms and to
show some impairment in functioning. Whether these individuals would be helped by the ready availability of psychiatric

services is a question to which many answers have been given, ranging from an enthusiastic affirmative to a contemptuous no. In any event, mental disorders, at least of the mild type, are extraordinarily widespread and are perhaps a concomitant of life in any society.

4 Social Class and Psychiatric Disorder

In the First Annual Report of the Registrar-General of Births, Deaths and Marriages in England, 1839, Dr William Farr remarked that:

The annual rate of mortality in some districts will be found to be 4 per cent, in others 2 per cent; in other words, the people in one set of circumstances live fifty years, while in another set of circumstances, which the registration will indicate, they do not live more than twenty-five years. In these wretched districts nearly 8 per cent are constantly sick, and the energy of the whole population is withered to the roots. Their arms are weak, their bodies wasted and their sensations embittered by privation and suffering. Half their life is passed in infancy, sickness and dependent helplessness ... while a part of the sickness is inevitable, and a part can only be expected to disappear before progressive social amelioration, a considerable proportion of the sickness and deaths may be suppressed by the general adoption of hygienic measures which are in actual but partial operation. It may be affirmed without great risk of exaggeration, that it is possible to reduce the annual deaths in England and Wales by 30,000 and to increase the vigour (may I not add the industry and wealth?) of the population in an equal proportion; for diseases are the iron index of misery, which recedes before strength, health and happiness as the mortality declines.

Class differentials in morbidity have not vanished even in the last third of the twentieth century. In addition to the differential distribution of diseases according to age, sex, race and place, the prevalence of disease also seems to vary in groups in terms of their style of life and their total environment. One convenient index of differing environment is socio-economic status or social class. Social class differences represent not only diverging occupations but divergence in education, speech, disposable income, physique, housing, nutrition, health care and innumerable other differences great and small.

The Decennial Survey of the General Register Office divides the population of England and Wales into five social classes primarily on the basis of occupation:

Class 1: The professional classes, made up of the higher professions, commissioned officers, company directors, bankers, and so forth.
Class 2: An intermediate class made up primarily of minor officials of public administration, proprietors of retail business, members of lower grade professions, clerks, farmers, teachers, etc.
Class 3: Composed of skilled workers.
Class 4: Partly skilled workers.
Class 5: Unskilled workers such as porters, builders, helpers, and so forth.

Prevalence rates of various diseases vary amongst the classes. For instance, rheumatic heart disease is higher in social class 5 than in social class 1 as are bronchitis, cancer of the stomach, tuberculosis, syphilis, hernia and accidents. On the other hand, cerebral vascular disease, appendicitis, suicide, gout and exophthalmic goitre appear to be more common amongst class 1 persons than in those of class 5. Infant mortality is consistently higher amongst the children of class 5 parents than in those of class 1. Data from elsewhere in the world seem to confirm the general proposition of class differentials in disease prevalence. However, just as was the case with the concept of mental illness, there are voices raised to dispute these findings. Kadushin (1964), an American sociologist, believes that any previously existing relationship between social class and the prevalence of illness is becoming weaker all the time and in many cases has disappeared. In his view, diseases are in the process of becoming homogeneously distributed within the classes. He feels that the explanation of previously observed class differentials lies in the realm of specific intervening variables such as malnutrition or poor health care, rather than being something specific to class *per se*. Consequently, as nutrition and public health improve, 'the gross factors which intervene between social class and the exposure to the disease will become more and more equal for all social classes'. There seems to be very little data to support this point of view. The overwhelming bulk of studies on illness and social class indicate there are still substantial differences in morbidity and mortality between the highest and the lowest classes.

One might presume that mental disorders also would not be immune to this class difference in distribution. There have been a number of studies in America and in the United Kingdom investigating the relationships between social class and mental illness. Most of these studies have involved attempts to establish a point prevalence of psychiatric morbidity for a defined population and then compare prevalence levels between social classes in the population.

Perhaps the most celebrated of these studies is that of Hollingshead and Redlich (1958) in New Haven, Connecticut, reported in their book, *Social Class and Mental Illness*. It is by far the most influential of all the studies and has been cited frequently in many different kinds of publications, both scientific and quasi-political, in order to bolster one or another point of view. The methods used in the study are representative of the best efforts of the interdisciplinary approach and the cautions and criticisms levelled at the methods and results are those which might apply to most epidemiological studies in social psychiatry.

The studies grew out of the collaboration of a sociologist, Professor Hollingshead, and a psychiatrist, Professor Redlich. As a fruit of their long conversations on the subject, two research questions emerged, namely: '(a) is mental illness related to class in our society? and (b) does a psychiatric patient's position in the status system affect how he is treated for his illness?' These research questions were formalized in a series of five hypotheses:

Hypothesis 1: The prevalence of treated mental illness is related significantly to an individual's position in the class structure.
Hypothesis 2: The types of diagnosed psychiatric disorders are connected significantly to the class structure.
Hypothesis 3: The kind of psychiatric treatment administered by

psychiatrists is associated with the patient's position in the class structure.

Hypothesis 4: Social and psychodynamic factors in the development of psychiatric disorders are correlative to an individual's position in the class structure.

Hypothesis 5: Mobility in the class structure is associated with the development of psychiatric difficulties.

The community chosen for the study was that of New Haven, Connecticut, the site of Yale University, at which institution both principal investigators held professorial appointments. In addition to the advantage of proximity, the size of the community, 240,000 at the time of the survey, was felt to be ideal for the purposes of the research in that it was large enough to insure confidentiality yet small enough for detailed studies. New Haven is also a community with a wide variety of differing subpopulations and a social structure which had been studied in great detail by sociologists over a period of time.

The various operations utilized in the study were subsumed under five categories:

1. The enumeration of individuals receiving psychiatric care.

2. A sample census of the general population.

3. The placement of the patient and the control populations in the class structure of the community.

4. Accumulation of detailed information about the practice of psychiatry.

5. Clinical study of fifty patients and their families included in the Control Case Study.

The first step was a psychiatric census of the defined population to establish a period prevalence and an incidence of identified cases. The definition of a case was: any person who was a resident of New Haven, West Haven, East Haven, North Haven, Hamden or Woodbridge, Connecticut, and who was in treatment with a psychiatrist or under the care of a psychiatric clinic or mental hospital between 31 May and 1

December 1950. The period prevalence so derived enumerated only medically identified cases and made no attempt to ascertain the prevalence of either untreated or unidentified mental illness in the community or to calculate mental illness under treatment by other than the medical profession. The incidence data related only to new cases coming into treatment during the study period.

There was a real problem in locating those individuals who should be enumerated. Complete enumeration obviously required the cooperation of a number of individuals and agencies, not only in the New Haven area but in other places as well because of the practice of some members of the community, particularly the well-to-do, of seeking psychiatric treatment elsewhere, notably in New York City. The necessity of achieving community cooperation in order to realize the objectives of any field survey is eminently worthy of mention at this point; careful diplomacy and unremitting work are necessary. It sounds quite simple to speak of enumerating all the cases in a given district but it turns out in practice to be extremely difficult, and often lengthy and tedious to obtain the actual and necessary information in accurate form.

The study progressed by compiling a list of (a) public, state and old people's hospitals, (b) clinics, (c) private hospitals and (d) private practitioners in Connecticut and adjacent areas. Depending upon the category of information wanted, institutions or practitioners in New York, New Hampshire, New Jersey, Rhode Island were also queried. In addition, famous psychiatric treatment centres from Canada to Florida and as far west as Topeka, Kansas, were also solicited to provide information about any New Haveners who might have travelled so far to obtain psychiatric treatment. After the lists were compiled a letter was carefully prepared, utilizing official stationery and the office and personal prestige of Professor Redlich to ensure its bona fides which explained the objectives of the census. Subsequently, a second letter was mailed to the various psychiatrists and institutions on the lists, and enclosed within it was an easy method of reply which also insured confidentiality. Prior to the mailing of the letters the principal medical investigator did an enormous amount of travelling and talking to such interested parties as superintendents of mental hospitals, directors of private and old people's hospitals, medical directors of clinics, psychiatric groups, and individual physicians in order to clarify the nature and importance of the study, and to ensure that the people whose cooperation would be requested understood that the investigators were serious and competent individuals, and that the study was a legitimate one which would be helpful in advancing the cause of good patient care. That this kind of public relations work is necessary has been shown by several abortive studies of mental retardation or mental illness, where the investigators failed to ensure the necessary community understanding and which therefore met with failure due to community opposition.

Where there was a failure to respond to written communications, Redlich personally telephoned the psychiatrists involved. Finally, a third letter was sent explaining that the initial enumeration was only a preamble to the psychiatric census. This letter indicated that each treatment agency reporting patients would be visited by members of the research team for interviews, during which a census schedule would be filled out on each patient. The principal features of the proposed interview were clarified and cooperation was solicited.

By means of this meticulous and intricate preparation, the investigators received the cooperation of all private and public hospitals, all clinics and all private practitioners save only two in Connecticut and nineteen in New York City, which was an excellent return rate.

After the preface to the study was over, schedules were prepared to develop and record the data of the psychiatric census. The interview schedule was divided into two parts: sociological and psychiatric. The sociological section recorded such demographic information as race, sex, age, occupation, education, place of birth, up-bringing, as well as social information such as a synopsis of the family history, national origin of the family and occupation of the parents. The psychiatric portion of the schedule listed such items as type of treatment and amount of payment given for treatment, the date of beginning treatment, the current treatment, number of past psychiatric hospitalizations, intensity and type of current and other previous therapy and diagnostic category. The data for each schedule were taken from the patient's clinical record by a sociologist and by a psychiatrist each separately searching the records for pertinent material to answer the questions in his own specialty. A check of abstractor reliability was carried out and it was found that reliability was very high, ranging on the sociological questions from 76 to 100 per cent and on the psychiatric ones from 79 to 96 per cent.

The diagnoses made by the patients' own psychiatrists were also checked for validity. The complete case record was examined by the team psychiatrists and then independently by two psychiatrists and a clinical psychologist before any case was rediagnosed. Although there were many disputed as to precise subcategory of diagnosis there were far fewer changes as to major category than had been originally anticipated. Seventeen per cent of the private practice cases needed to be rediagnosed and less than 6 per cent of the hospital and clinic cases.

In order to compare directly the characteristics of patients v. non-patients by class position, data of a demographic and social nature had to be gathered on the general population resident in the area covered by the psychiatric census. A 5 per cent sample of the households in this area was enumerated. Individual households were selected because they were the primary type of dwelling within the community rather than blocks of flats, for example. In any type of census operation there are many people who are either difficult to find and count or who pose a methodological problem as to whether they should be counted at all. For example, in this study the investigators did not count such individuals as students resident in college, prisoners in jail, patients in general hospitals or hotel dwellers, although other kinds of surveys with different goals might well have counted them. The census takers used the City Directory of the City of New Haven and randomly selected 3383 household addresses plus 225 households known to be located in the poorest areas of the city. The interviewers were generally students in Yale University or their wives who were specially trained for the purpose of the study. Less than 5 per cent of the households refused to cooperate. Information relating to age, sex, race, occupation, education, marital status, religion, economic status and whether or not the household was owned or rented was gathered. Both the patients enumerated in the psychiatric census and the respondents contacted in the 5 per cent sample were categorized as to social class, utilizing an index of social position constructed by Professor Hollingshead. Essentially, the index was a weighted scale utilizing the respondent's (or the patient's) occupation, education and his 'ecological area of residence' to determine his social position. The location of the household was analysed according to a residential scale based on early work in the New Haven community. The individual's occupation was scored by a system which was a modification of the system used in classifying occupations into socio-economic groups by the United States Bureau of the Census. The educational scale had seven positions ranging from less than seven years of school to the highest graduate professional training. According to the investigators the index had as its premises three assumptions:

1. That social stratification exists in the community.

2. That status positions are determined mainly by a few commonly accepted cultural characteristics.

3. That items symbolic of status may be scaled and combined by the use of the statistical procedures so that a researcher can quickly, reliably and meaningfully stratify the population.

Utilizing these criteria, 3·4 per cent of the community's population was placed in class 1, which in New Haven meant a well-to-do, well-educated group, all Caucasian, and primarily Protestant. In the main, this subpopulation represented old New England families, who were the community's professional and business elite with income, dwellings and social life to match.

Nine per cent of the community was placed into social class 2. Class 2 was composed primarily of managers and lesser ranking professionals, almost all of whom had some formal education beyond high school and who were reasonably affluent. More than half of this group was Protestant and 'striving for success' was felt to be particularly marked in this category. Social class 3 comprised 21·4 per cent of the community's population. This class contained individuals who were engaged in salaried administrative and clerical pursuits, technicians, supervisors in factories, or owners of small businesses. The majority of this group were Roman Catholics and were descendents of recent immigrants to the United States. Social class 4 represented 48·5 per cent of the community. This group contained the skilled workers and lower rank clerical and sales workers. The majority of the members of this class had less than a high school education. Only 7 per cent of the individuals in this group came from 'old Yankee families'.

Class 5 comprised 17·7 per cent of the households. This group included the low-paid unskilled or semi-skilled workers with low income, poor education and slum dwelling. In this category there were many different kinds of family constellations, very little reading, a deep-seated distrust of authority, a necessity of living for the moment, coupled with a very hard struggle for existence in poorly paid and unskilled jobs.

Finally, the census investigations were supplemented by a controlled case study in which fifty patients, twenty-five psychoneurotics and twenty-five schizophrenics, were selected from social classes 3 and 5 for an exhaustive study both of a clinical and social nature. Detailed data on each patient was obtained. The patients were all Caucasian between the ages of twenty-two and forty-four. The patients were interviewed as well as their therapists and their families. In addition, their clinical records were examined and Professor Redlich saw each patient personally.

This outline gives some notion of the enormous amount of effort and care which had to go into the construction of the study and the gathering of the necessary information.

Following the enumeration of patients by the psychiatric

census and the delineation of the social and demographic characteristics of both the patient group and the non-patient comparison population, the investigators utilized the data to test their original hypotheses. The first three hypotheses were supported by the data. The principal finding was that the lower the social class the greater was the proportion of treated patients in the population, although this statement needs qualification (see Table 5). For example, the upper class, class

Table 5 Class Status and the Distribution of Patients and Non-Patients in the Population

	Population per cent	
Class	Patients	Non-patients
1	1·0	3·0
2	7·0	8·4
3	13·7	20·4
4	40·1	49·8
5	38·2	18·4
	$n = 1891$	236,940

$\chi^2 = 509·81, 4 \text{ d.f.}, p < 0·001$

Source: Hollingshead and Redlich (1958, pt 3, ch. 7, p. 199)

1, which had 3 per cent of the population had only 1 per cent of the patients. Class 2 had 8·4 per cent of the population and only 7 per cent of the patients. Class 3 had 20 per cent of the total population and 13·7 per cent of the patients. Class 4 had 49·8 per cent of the population and 40 per cent of the patients. On the other hand, class 5 comprised 18·4 per cent of the general population yet it contained 38·2 per cent of the patients. If one analysed the data for rate, then class 5 had about three times the rate of treated psychoses than did classes 1 and 2. A glance at the table indicates that the main problem resides in class 5 since the other four classes have only modest differences between their total population and the prevalence of treated psychiatric patients. Therefore, the major finding is that the lowest class had a very much greater rate of identified psychiatric disorder than did all the other classes.

The authors conclude that their first hypothesis, that is, that the prevalence of treated mental illness is related significantly to an individual's position in the class structure, may be regarded as substantiated. If the measure of incidence, that is, new cases coming into treatment, were used instead of prevalence, the class differentials remained. Once again, the class 5 individuals had higher incidence rates than did the other classes.

As regards hypothesis 2, which spoke to the relationship of types of psychiatric disorders to class structure, the data indicated that what was true for the overall rate of mental illness was even more striking when psychoses (principally schizophrenia) were considered alone. The distribution of neurotic illnesses was much more complicated than the distribution of psychoses. There appeared to be 'class-typed neuroses' with sociopathic disturbances tending to occur in the lowest class and anxiety reactions in the middle class. The neurotic disturbances of the upper two classes were characterized by individual dissatisfaction with self or life accomplishments.

The data confirmed in the most striking way the third hypothesis, namely that the nature of treatment given to a patient depends very much on his position in the class structure. Prolonged psychotherapy and psychoanalysis were given almost exclusively in the upper classes. Organic therapies, such as electric shock, rather than prolonged psychotherapy tended to be given most often to neurotics in social classes 3 and 4. In the psychotic group the class 5 patients were found to become chronic state hospital patients in disproportionate numbers. The bulk of these patients received electro-shock therapy. In terms of percentages, the authors divided treatment into three categories: psychotherapy of some type which 32 per cent of the patients received; organic treatments of one type or another which 31·7 per cent of the patients received; and custodial care without specific treatment which 36·3 per cent of the patients received. The class differences in type of therapy received are graphically shown in Table 6.

Table 6 Distribution of the Principal Types of Therapy by Social Class

Social class	Psychotherapy		Organic therapy		No treatment	
	number	per cent	number	per cent	number	per cent
1	14	73.7	2	10.5	3	15.8
2	107	81.7	15	11.4	9	6.9
3	136	52.7	74	28.7	48	18.6
4	237	31.1	288	37.1	242	31.8
5	115	16.1	234	32.7	367	51.2

$\chi^2 = 336.58, p < 0.001$
Source: Hollingshead and Redlich (1953)

In 1968 Myers and Bean published a book entitled *A Decade Later: A Follow-up of Social Class and Mental Illness* in which these authors detailed the results of a follow-up study of the same New Haven population. The follow-up study showed again that social-class status did carry with it an inference about clinical course of psychiatric illnesses in the various classes. The lower-class patients, in contrast to the upper-class ones, tended either to stay in hospital continuously or to be readmitted more readily if released so that the public and old people's hospitals had a disproportionate share of lower class people resident in them at any one time. It was found that amongst the non-hospitalized, the upper-class patients tended to have greater psychological impairment than those from the lowest classes. However, the former presumably lived and worked in environments which are more tolerant of eccentricities than would be the environment of an unskilled worker.

We might sum up the results of this landmark study, which has occasioned so much discussion and, indeed, modification of psychiatric thinking, by stating that mental illness of a treated nature, particularly psychoses, is not uniformly distributed amongst the social classes but rather that the lowest class tends to have a disproportionate share of the identified illness. Secondly, the treatment given for mental illness in various social classes varies, with higher classes tending to receive more psychotherapy and intensive treatment and the lower classes more custodial care. Long-term follow-up indicates that class differentials continue to affect the patients' clinical course even at the present when, subsequent to the time of the initial psychiatric census, powerful psychopharmacological agents have been introduced.

In the final phase of the research, the investigators used the previously mentioned intensive case study of fifty patients in an attempt to gather data relevant to hypotheses 4 and 5. Hypothesis 4 dealt with the social and psychodynamic features of each class within the social structure which might be associated with psychiatric illness. Hypothesis 5 concerned social mobility and mental health. Striking differences were found in the amount and type of external stresses to which class 3 as opposed to class 5 individuals were subjected. Extreme differences in family life, family communication, attitudes towards mental illness, attitudes towards treatment, and indeed in most aspects of life were documented.

A propos of hypothesis 5, social mobility did seem in some instances to be associated with emotional problems. The authors distinguished two subtypes of the (upwardly) mobile: first, the climber 'who appears to actually move up the social ladder' à la Becky Sharp, and 'the strainer' who tries hard but does not succeed. In both instances, upward striving was associated with considerable anxiety, guilt and often psychosomatic symptoms in those playing this game. Such climbers appeared to have certain unpleasant character traits of the type which made life difficult for those about them. The second major type of socially mobile person is, of course, the one who is falling downward on the social scale. Generally such individuals are caught up with problems revolving around alcohol or drug addiction. Their self-destructive and depressed behaviour make them particularly difficult patients to handle.

When speaking of downward mobility one must mention the pioneering study of Faris and Dunham (1939) entitled *Mental Disorders in Urban Areas: An Ecological Study of*

Schizophrenia and Other Psychoses, in which it was established that there were great differences in the patterns of mental hospital admission rates for psychoses in various census tracts in Chicago. Certain deteriorated and slum areas in the central city, particularly those in which there were resident a high number of transient and rootless people of the lower classes, had the most elevated rates. These high hospitalization rates were concentrated in and around the central business districts with rates declining in every direction toward the periphery. A dweller in the central city was fifteen times more likely to be committed to a mental hospital than was a person living in the outskirts of Chicago. Some social scientists and psychiatrists on viewing these data advanced the hypothesis of 'downward drift'. The main thrust of this idea is that the individuals living in these deteriorated ecological areas of shabby lodgings, down-at-heel hotels and ruined tenements were individuals who became mentally ill in better circumstances and then drifted downward both in social class and in area of residence to end up concentrated in these unfortunate districts.

Hollingshead and Redlich attempted to answer this question by checking the residential histories of 428 patients who had lived in New Haven all their lives. The conclusion was reached that virtually all the members of class 1 and 2 patient groups had always lived in the best areas of New Haven and the members of class 5 had always lived in the slum and, therefore, there was no evidence of a significant 'drift' up or down in the patients themselves. Their data thus supported the original thought of Faris and Dunham themselves that the downward drift hypothesis did not account for their findings.

In contrast to the findings of Hollingshead and Redlich, Goldberg and Morrison (1963) working at the MRC Social Medicine Research Unit, London, conducted a documentary and clinical study of schizophrenia and social class which brought forward strong evidence to support the notion of downward drift. They first studied a national sample of males age twenty-five to thirty-four admitted for the first time to mental hospitals in England and Wales. They classified these first admissions by social class and confirmed the usual finding of an excessive representation of social class 5 patients. The social class system of categories used was that of the Registrar General's, with class 5 representing primarily unskilled labourers. When they examined the social class of the fathers of the patients at the time of patients' birth, they found that the fathers' class distribution was essentially that of the population as a whole and not concentrated in class 5. A complementary clinical study of a representative series of male schizophrenics age fifteen to thirty living in outer London also showed a decline in occupational status from father to son. This finding was confirmed by careful examination of the patients' own histories which indicated that although a patient might begin as the child of a class 1 or 2 parents, say, attending a grammar school or even a minor public school, he gradually showed evidence of increasing failure in life and drifted downward to end up working at an unskilled or at the best, a semi-skilled occupation. The authors attributed this discrepancy between the success of the father and of the son to the process of the schizophrenic illness itself which so often seriously interferes with the patient's ability to get on in life. This interference seemed most marked in the lives of patients from the highest and from the lowest social class. For instance, those class 1 or 2 patients who attempted to achieve a university education or to run a business met with disaster and those who began life as children of unskilled workers also had very great difficulties. In the case of the former the high demands implicit in the educational or occupational situations proved too much for their brittle emotional resources. In the case of the latter, the nature of unskilled work and the thin margin on which unskilled workers live apparently did not afford sufficient support to such individuals when even partially psychotic and they tended to drop out of the labour market entirely and remain in hospital. In contrast, patients from social classes 3 and 4 often managed to carry on in their skilled trades in spite of a history of psychosis.

The Goldberg and Morrison study is not directly comparable to that of Hollingshead and Redlich because the Hollingshead and Redlich findings refer mainly to chronic patients in mental hospitals and not exclusively to first admissions. As previously noted, the class 5 patients tended to remain in hospital over the long term and it may be that even amongst them, the patients who remained in hospital came primarily from a class 5 family origin. The whole question is surely moot and it seems as if studies with contrasting findings could be matched *ad infinitum*. For example, Lystad (1957) in New Orleans, and Gerard and Houston (1953) in Worchester, Massachusetts, found evidence for mobility and drift whereas Clausen and Kohn (1959) in Hagerstown, Maryland, and Turner and Wagenfeld (1967) in upstate New York did not.

Since social class or, as it is called in some studies, 'socio-economic status' does seem to be associated with the differential prevalence of mental illness, the question arises as to whether this association implies any sort of causation. Does being born and brought up in a lower-class family predispose one to the development of mental illness to a greater degree than would be the case if one had a higher-class origin? For example, it might be that the style of family life in the slums would exert a lasting and deleterious effect on mental health. Halliday published his work *Psychosocial Medicine* (1948) which dealt with the interrelationships of psychosomatic disease incidence and changing patterns of life, including patterns of child rearing. For example, he saw a vast difference between child-rearing patterns of the 1870s and those of the 1930s. The nineteenth-century pattern was one of virtually universal breast feeding, late toilet training and minimal fussing over the child. There was, of course, an unhygienic environment from the standpoint of bacterial disease; however, he felt that the psychological climate for the infant was very good and allowed a natural unfolding of development. In the 1930s breast feeding was less common, early toilet training was the rule, houses were furnished in such a way that there were many dangerous objects such as electric sockets which did not exist a hundred years before, perambulators were commonly used, families were smaller and much more was expected of the infant in the way of performance. In Halliday's mind this type of child rearing created an 'imposed system of conditioning which prematurely provoked, or predisposed to, bodily disorders by inducing tensional states of dysfunctions in the gastro-intestinal tract, the respiratory system, the cardiovascular system, the voluntary muscular system, and so on', and which might account, at least in part, for changing patterns of psychosomatic disorders, for example, the sharp increase in the incidence of peptic ulcers in men noted in the twentieth century.

Similarly, there are many investigators who believe that disordered family relationships and distorted intrafamilial communications during childhood play a strong etiological role in the genesis of psychoses such as schizophrenia. Lidz (1963) and his colleagues at Yale University as well as Wynne and Singer (1963) of the US National Institute of Mental Health are prominent amongst researchers who have consistently demonstrated bizarre interactional patterns in the families of schizophrenic patients. They have compared these disordered families with families containing mentally normal children and have shown gross differences in all dimensions of family life, including such areas as decision making, privacy, communications, punishment, reward, mutual gratification, incestuous behaviour and so forth. It could be that such disturbed families are, in fact, more common in social class 5 than in the other classes. Infancy and childhood in many lower-class families might be characterized by stormy and loveless relationships, severe conflicts and broken homes, all of which might promote defects of ego, conscience and character. The vicissitudes of adolescence in the slums might exacerbate intrafamilial tensions and indeed it is in late adolescence that the onset of schizophrenia is most common. In addition to family problems in the lower classes, it might be that the surrounding environment with its endemic economic difficulties, few community supports, low cohesiveness, high crime prevalence, easy availability of drugs and other malevolent social features might predispose to the development of mental illness. For example, in work at the MRC Social Medicine Research Unit, Power (personal communication, 1967), a research social worker, has indicated that even among boys of homogeneous social origin in the London borough of Tower Hamlets there was an enormous discrepancy in juvenile delinquency rates between certain schools in the district. This was true even among schools which seemed to serve precisely the same type of population. These data indicated that a certain kind of psychopathological phenomenon, namely, anti-social behaviour, might be profoundly affected by proximate environmental variables. On the other hand, it is rather difficult to see how such general aspects of life such as poverty or social isolation in the slums eventuate in the offspring of certain families developing relatively specific syndromes such as paranoid schizophrenia or manic-depressive psychosis. Studies have demonstrated that the poor have a very large number of bodily complaints not always related to organic disease but, even so, overt psychosis is by no means a ubiquitous phenomenon even amongst the families of the poorest and most depressed districts.

We have seen how environmental agents such as educational or economic deprivation, or pathological styles of child rearing, or tangled intrafamilial communication have been postulated as explanations of the apparent increased prevalence of serious mental disorders in the lowest socio-economic classes. Others have considered the possibility of some genetic explanation for this phenomena, to wit, that the low social and economic position of the patient or his family is a result of his mental disease rather than the cause of it. Adherents of this viewpoint have considered serious mental disorders of a psychotic nature, including both schizophrenia and depressive illnesses, to be primarily organic diseases of the brain of an inherited nature. They have argued that the lowest social class contains a disproportionate number of families carrying this kind of genetic constitution or predisposition. Hence, there would be a perpetuation of a high incidence of the disorders in this class even in the absence of facilitating environmental variables. An underlying presumption would be that at some point in the history of each slum family predisposed to psychosis there had existed a progenitor who had fallen into this class by reason of his lack of normal mental facilities (downward drift again). In this theoretical position, it is thought that the adverse effects of a life of poverty, including such factors as poor nutrition with its stifling effect on brain development as well as malignant psychic stresses, might merely enhance the inherited predisposition to severe mental illness.

A study by Heston and Denney (1968) in Oregon did indicate that the children of schizophrenic mothers, even if reared completely apart from those mothers, showed a greater tendency to develop schizophrenia later than did a comparison group of children from foundling homes reared apart from their non-schizophrenic mothers.

There have been many other ingenious explanations postulated to elucidate the association of psychosis and low status. However, certain critics have thought the finding to be an artefact resulting from various methodological faults in the studies rather than being a valid association. These possible methodological flaws in the studies of one serious mental disease, schizophrenia, are considered at length in the incisive review by Mishler and Scotch (1963) of Harvard University. Others have also dilated on this topic.

Suffice it to say that there may be class biases in hospital admissions and in the diagnostic process as well as errors in the measurement of socio-economic status. Physicians may tend to give the diagnosis of psychosis more readily to a lower-class person than to an upper-class one and, in turn, may be more reluctant to release a lower-class patient back into his impoverished community than they would be to release a middle-class one to a supportive environment. In a similar vein, it has been shown that respondents may give different answers to the same questions depending on the identity of the person administering the questionnaire. For example, an interviewer of a different race or sex from the respondent may elicit a different answer than would an interviewer of the same sex and race. In addition, the use of prevalence rates rather than incidence rates makes for great difficulties in the interpretation of correlations between variables. This is particularly true in the major mental diseases because of their great tendency towards chronicity and thus towards increasing prevalence. We have already seen how lower-class patients tend to become chronic residents in hospital and this would be reflected in any hospital prevalence study. On the other hand, upper-class patients tend to be released to the community even if they retain considerable manifestations of mental illness. Once returned to the community they might not be counted as a case in a prevalence study. What one really needs to know is the true incidence rate in the various classes. Hollingshead and Redlich attempted to do this but, of course, their data were based solely on identified cases and it is by no means proved that the data represented any sort of true incidence rate. Goldberg and Morrison also used hospitalized cases only. Nevertheless the data from so many sources, including pioneering work in the United Kingdom by Hare (1956) and Cooper (1961), have indicated the relative excess of psychotic diseases, as measured by hospitalization, in individuals of the lowest socio-economic status.

It should be emphasized that social class is by no means a unitary variable. The dimensions and meaning of social class are at least as controversial a topic as that of psychiatric diagnosis. Not only are there controversies about methods of gauging social class, that is, whether to use occupation, income, education, residence, accent or type of school attended, but there are also disputes as to the significance of type of schooling, or how to gauge the ancestral family's social class and so forth. In addition to the problems of deciding about what markers to use there is the question about what social class encompasses. Certainly it implies more than the stark facts of the indices used to distinguish the various groups. Rather, class involves so many vast differences in style of life both of an obvious and a subtle nature as to make one certain that it should have its effect on mental disease as it so clearly does on normal mental life, emotionality and conduct. The rub is to distinguish what specific variables within the vast complex of lower-class, middle-class or upper-class life styles might be responsible for some particular disease outcome. No investigations have come really close to this goal. The discussions about interaction of a class style of life with manifestations of mental disease contain an extraordinarily high proportion of speculation and rather scanty hard data.

To summarize, there have been a number of studies over many decades about the relationship of mental illness and social class. It would appear from these studies, which utilize primarily but not exclusively prevalence figures of identified psychiatric cases compared to a described population, that there is an excess accumulation of patients with psychotic mental disease in the lowest socio-economic class, that is, the class consisting of unskilled labourers and unemployed slum dwellers. The point may be regarded, however, as not completely proven because of the methodological difficulties involved in the use of prevalence rates and in the possible artefacts introduced by diagnostic and therapeutic bias and error, and by methodological problems involved in the definition of the population at risk and its class structure. Those who regard this excess accumulation phenomenon as real rather than artefactual have advanced various hypotheses to explain it. These explanations include the notion of downward drift, either on the part of the enumerated patient or his progenitors, and with an accumulation in the lowest class of families which contain the genetic propensity for the development of psychotic mental illness, the pathogenic effects on the developing psyche of the social, psychological and economic stresses and strains of family life in the slums.

5 Social Factors in the Onset of Disease

Only scientific physicians have ever doubted that events in life influence the start of disease. The laity has always been sure that people do die of broken hearts and that the onset of illness in humans is facilitated by the vicissitudes of life – great and small. The celebrated Swiss-American psychiatrist, Adolph Meyer (1950–52), although trained originally as a neuropathologist, was among the pioneers in an attempt to translate this folk wisdom into a more systematic observational framework. He developed the 'life chart' which was essentially a schema into which the major events of a patient's life could be placed in such a way as to display their progression graphically and in juxtaposition to the major diseases that had arisen during the course of the patient's life. Meyer emphasized the importance of 'changes of habitat, school entrance, graduations or changes or failures, the various jobs, the dates of possibly important births and deaths in the family, and other fundamentally important environmental influences' in the facilitation of the onset of disease. Meyer did his work primarily in the early decades of this century. Subsequent work of a physiological nature by Cannon, Selye, Wolff, and many others, have suggested mechanisms by which social events could profoundly influence the inner state through complex neuro-endocrinological pathways.

In the field of psychiatry there has always been a lively interest in those events which seem to be linked with the onset of mental illness, particularly of an acute type. In this connection, there are several classical expositions which have been put forward to illuminate disease onset.

Perhaps the most famous of these are the speculations of Karl Abraham (1912) and Sigmund Freud (1917) about the onset of depressive illness. Their essential argument is that pathological depression might be usefully compared with normal grief. In both cases the individual has suffered some sort of loss. In its most obvious form the loss would be the death of a close relative. In the case of normal grief there is a gradual working through of the pain associated with the loss and a resumption of normal activities and normal feelings. However, the individual predisposed to depression retains his grief following a loss for an abnormally lengthy period. The grief is of pathological character and duration and is heavily intermixed with extreme feelings of guilt. The explanation of this guilt and melancholy is postulated to be extreme hostility of an unconscious nature which was directed towards the dead person, who had been symbolically introjected or incorporated into the patient's own psyche at some earlier point of time so that the unconscious hatred that the patient had for the lost person is now directed towards the patient himself.

Since the early part of the twentieth century when Abraham and Freud put forward these notions there have been many criticisms and modifications of their original ideas. For example, loss is now interpreted in a less literal sense and can mean not only the death of a near relative but all manner of symbolic losses of esteem due to such things as being fired from a position, failure to be promoted, being arrested and so forth. Theories regarding the onset of depression which lay emphasis on social and psychological phenomena are not necessarily incompatible with the modern biochemical theories of depression since all effects of social phenomena would have to be mediated through the mechanism of the brain and its biochemical constituents.

Schmale and his co-worker Engel (1967) have suggested the possibility of a very high incidence of recent object loss and depressive reactions even amongst an unselected medical population. They have felt that a 'giving up/given up' complex is a precursor of disease onset. Essentially this complex involves the patient's own perception of himself and represents his own sense of loss about which he can do nothing. This feeling of threatened or actual loss is, of course, occasioned by social events in the patient's life. For example, the loss of the family home because of urban redevelopment or the loss of the patient's business because of successful competition on the part of a new supermarket might set in motion a train of events which lead to illness onset. When such an event occurs in an individual predisposed to the development of this complex and subsequent illness, certain characteristic features appear. There is a plethora of feelings of helplessness, that is, firstly a sense of environmental deprivation and secondly a sense of hopelessness, in which the individual feels that he cannot overcome the effects of this environmental loss because of his own personal inadequacies and failings. Both feelings may be present in the same individual or one or the other may vastly predominate. In any case the patient perceives himself as less competent, less in control, less gratified, less secure than in the past. During this time he sees the external environment as being threatenly different from the expectations of the past, he experiences marked discontinuities and envisages a bleak future. This troubled period is likely to revive in him feelings, memories and behaviour connected with past difficulties.

It is postulated that there are three major pathways into which a person who has developed a 'giving up/given up' complex as the result of some environmental deprivation may turn. Firstly, the individual may develop new and better means of coping with his troubles or happily the environment may change to his advantage in which case he can resume his former level of adjustment. Secondly, he may become physically ill; or thirdly, he may become either psychiatrically ill or socially deviant. A number of ingenious studies have been done by Schmale and Engel to test these notions, utilizing both patient and non-patient populations. The studies have been primarily retrospective in character and while they have brought forward evidence to substantiate these hypotheses, once again the matter may be regarded as not yet completely proven.

In an attempt to put into objective and quantitative terms the intensity of various life stresses and the relationship between these stresses and disease onset, Professor Thomas Holmes of the University of Washington, Seattle, and Dr Richard Rahe (1967) of the US Navy Medical Neuropsychiatric Research Unit, San Diego, California, have developed devices to gauge the magnitude of social events in the production of life change. The events enumerated pertain to major areas of significance in the social aspects of human life. The scale was originally developed on Americans and American families; however, studies abroad have indicated that there are many similarities of human life which extend through all cultures and which are viewed by all nationalities tested as having essentially the same magnitude of impact (see Table 7).

Table 7 Social Readjustment Rating Scale

Rank	Life event	Mean value
1	Death of spouse	100
2	Divorce	73
3	Marital separation	65
4	Jail term	63
5	Death of close family member	63
6	Personal injury or illness	53
7	Marriage	50
8	Fired at work	47
9	Marital reconciliation	45
10	Retirement	45
11	Change in health of family member	44
12	Pregnancy	40
13	Sex difficulties	39
14	Gain of new family member	39
15	Business readjustment	39
16	Change in financial state	38
17	Death of close friend	37
18	Change to different line of work	36
19	Change in number of arguments with spouse	35
20	Mortgage over $10,000	31
21	Foreclosure of mortgage or loan	30
22	Change in responsibilities at work	29

Rank	Life event	Mean value
23	Son or daughter leaving home	29
24	Trouble with in-laws	29
25	Outstanding personal achievement	28
26	Wife begins or stops work	26
27	Begin or end school	26
28	Change in living conditions	25
29	Revision of personal habits	24
30	Trouble with boss	23
31	Change in work hours or conditions	20
32	Change in residence	20
33	Change in schools	20
34	Change in recreation	19
35	Change in church activities	19
36	Change in social activities	18
37	Mortgage or loan less than $10,000	17
38	Change in sleeping habits	16
39	Change in number of family get-togethers	15
40	Change in eating habits	15
41	Vacation	13
42	Christmas	12
43	Minor violations of the law	11

Source: Holmes and Rahe (1967, p. 216)

The life events utilized in the scale included such areas as occupation, residence, economics, recreation, religion, family and social relationships. Each of these events either was indicative of or required a significant change in the ongoing life pattern of the individual, without regard to its possible psychological or symbolic significance. Many of the events were not intrinsically adverse in type but all involved some impingement on the steady state of the individual's life.

The method of psychophysics was used as a model for the construction of this scale. In psychophysics the psychological perception of the quality, quantity, magnitude and intensity of physical phenomena are studied. The individual's subjective assessment is compared with the physical dimension being perceived, for example, the length of the rod, the loudness of a sound or the brightness of a light. Such psychophysical studies have shown a certain lawfulness in the human perception of physical phenomena. Similarly, in an attempt to quantify the impact of life events on an individual's coping mechanisms, the assumption was made that there would be a convergence amongst people involving quantitative judgements about psychosocial phenomena. Indeed, this optimism was justified. As indicated in Table 7, experiments conducted among several American subgroups, as well as Japanese, Swedes and Danes, have shown that agreement was high regardless of factors such as age, sex, marital status, education, social class, race, nationality and religion.

Initially, the subjects were told that a single item, namely marriage, was to be assigned an arbitrary score, say fifty points. They were then asked to rate as compared to marriage, the amount of turmoil, upheaval and social readjustment necessitated by events such as death of a spouse, divorce, trouble with the boss, detention in jail, foreclosure on a mortgage, death of a close friend, change in residence, promotion, demotion, changing occupations and so forth, to a total of forty-three different events. As was previously stated, there was a high degree of concensus amongst the respondents as to the relative impact of these various events.

Having thus empirically developed a scaling device to assess the magnitude of life events, the investigators utilized this instrument in an attempt to predict health change. The underlying hypothesis was that those individuals who during a given period of time, say a one or two-year period, who had a very high life crisis score, indicating a large number of life changes packed into a short span of time, would be more likely to develop a major health change than those individuals who had a low life crisis score during the same epoch, indicating a relatively tranquil period with little demands on the coping mechanisms of the body.

Studies utilizing the life crisis scale have been carried out on a wide variety of populations and have tended to confirm the basic hypothesis. In Navy populations, Rahe, Arthur and

Gunderson (1971) obtained life crisis scores on the entire crews of various naval vessels prior to their being deployed either to the Far East or to the Mediterranean. After a period of six months the crews and their health records were re-examined and the correlation between life crisis score and health change was noted. Those sailors who fell in the highest decile for a life crisis score, that is, who had a maximum amount of unsettling life events in the year prior to the cruise, developed twice as much illness as did that portion of the crew in the lowest decile. Although these predictions related to the entire gamut of illnesses, it is also clear that there is a greater risk of developing mental as well as physical illness following a period of great psychosocial stress than following one of an uneventful nature.

Of course, the social forces of the type just enumerated are ubiquitous ones and appear as stressors in the lives of all humans who reach adult life. However, there are certain general upheavals of society which may embrace an entire nation or continent and provide a general raising of the total level of demand on individuals, although, of course, even in total war some people are less roughly handled than are others by circumstance. Two of the most obvious and overwhelming social stresses are war and incarceration in a concentration camp. It will be of interest to discuss the effects on mental health of both of these phenomena.

The effects of the Second World War on civilian rates of admission to mental hospitals was, if anything, to cause them to decline. Data from Norway, France, Belgium and the United Kingdom all showed either a reduction or no significant increase in admission rates, particularly for psychoses. In the United States, however, during that same period there was a significant increase in the rate of first admissions to mental hospitals amongst males, particularly between the ages of twenty and thirty, an increase that was not seen in females. In addition, while the mental hospital admission rate in Europe might have declined during the war, there was some evidence to suggest that such psychoneurotic disorders as anxiety reactions and such psychosomatic diseases as perforated peptic ulcer increased, particularly in civilian populations exposed to aerial bombing.

In the US and UK armed forces there appeared to be a definite increase in total psychiatric admission rates during the First and Second World Wars and the Korean War (for the US forces) as compared to peacetime service. It was previously mentioned that the rates for psychoses seemed to vary little in war time; however, the rates for psychoneurotic disorders did show a marked increase and there have been delineated, beginning in the First World War, a series of specific psychiatric syndromes associated with combat. These syndromes were probably little noted prior to the First World War although there is some mention of them in connection with the Russo–Japanese War of 1904–5. Apart from the probability that these disorders were overlooked by previous observers, it is also true that prior to the First World War most battles lasted several days at the most and there were few campaigns indeed which lasted year after bloody year as was the case on the Western Front in the First World War. There was essentially four years of virtually continuous fighting from 1914 to 1918, a catastrophe totally unprecedented in the history of mankind. No one can doubt the extraordinary and lifelong effects of perpetual bombardment, disease, filth, insomnia and stress on men of even the slightest sensitivity. The travail of the men in the trenches has been well chronicled by writers such as Robert Graves (1929) and Siegfried Sassoon (1930). One can imagine hundreds of thousands of men who would have been able to withstand the one day stress of a Waterloo, but who went under after several months of being in the lines in Flanders. Such cases were labelled as 'shell shock' during the First World War and 'combat fatigue' during the Second. Initially it was thought that the concussive effects of near misses by artillery directly affected the brain in such a way as to bring about the characteristic signs; however, it gradually became apparent that the causes of this syndrome were multiple and much more complex than simple trauma. Physical factors such as insomnia, poor nutrition, thermal stress and perhaps even exhaustion of the neuro-endocrine axis by continuous and overwhelming stress played some part in the development of symptoms. In addition, there were many psychosocial factors operative in the incidence of mental breakdown in combat. Units in which there was high morale based on confidence in the leadership, in the abilities of one's comrades and in the effectiveness of one's weapons had a much lower incidence of psychological breakdown than did units in which there was no confidence in victory, no confidence in leadership, and mistrust between the men. Early in the combat situation, many men utilized the psychic defence of denial: the feeling that they were personally invulnerable to the death and destruction that struck others. This feeling inevitably disappeared as the combat experience continued.

Some soldiers, of course, develop during the combat situation psychoses or psychoneuroses of the type seen commonly in civil life, that is, they may become schizophrenic, depressed or phobic without any necessary relationship to the military environment. However, the majority of men who experience an emotional breakdown during combat fall into a well-defined symptom complex with both acute and chronic phases. The principal manifestations are simply exaggerations of symptoms being shown by most of the soldiers in combat. These include severe insomnia, recurrent nightmares, anorexia, trembling, irritability, tachycardia, gastro-intestinal symptoms, numbness and tingling of the extremities, careless exposure to enemy fire and severe reactions to battlefield noises.

In no other area of psychiatry is the relationship between endopsychic and social forces so graphically illustrated. There is an extreme range of vulnerability to combat stress ranging from those individuals of great predisposition (usually ones with a long history of emotional conflict and neurotic problems) to individuals with enormous ego strength. It is a battlefield truism that 'every man has his breaking point'. This statement may also be true although there are some people who seem to be virtually invulnerable to environmental vicissitudes; however, in the vast majority of cases, individuals subjected to very severe and prolonged combat stress develop a full-blown combat syndrome. On the other hand, social forces not only include the morale and cohesiveness of the man's military unit, alluded to in a preceding paragraph, but also to medical administrative policy. For example, in the early stages of both the First and Second World Wars psychiatrists in the American armed forces tended to send all combat fatigue cases immediately to the rear areas for further evacuation to the USA. The psychiatric casualty rate rapidly grew to intolerable populations. In 1918 (and again after rediscovery in 1943!) the principle of treating casualties as close to the front as possible was adopted. This administrative decision proved able to halt the upward trend of psychiatric losses which if continued would have effectively crippled the armed forces. Psychiatrists were stationed at the divisional level and psychiatric treatment stations were established relatively close to the front line. It was found that by treating patients in these locations, regression to chronic invalidism, which had been seen in the majority of cases evacuated in the past, was largely prevented. Men who had been evacuated to the homeland while their units were still in a combat situation often developed a pervasive sense of grief and guilt about leaving their units and their comrades after the initial relief of escape had worn off. This guilt might be very chronic and persistent.

In the chronic phases of the combat syndrome the patient might show continuing psychosomatic disorders, continuing nightmares, pervasive anxiety, restriction of interest and intellectual activity and occasional outbursts of aggressive rage. Patients might also show obsessive compulsive features such as the need for particular ceremonial actions before they felt able to eat or sleep or even to walk about.

All authorities agree that the most important feature of the treatment of acute combat syndrome is the prevention of chronicity. Once established in a chronic pattern the patient proves to be extraordinarily resistant to rehabilitative efforts. On the other hand, the vast majority of acute cases can be prevented from entering a chronic stage. During the period after war, it appears that compensation, particularly in the form of a very small but permanent pension, is probably antitherapeutic. Individuals who have such pensions do seem to be extraordinarily resistant to occupational and social restoration and it is felt that this practice tends to hold the patient in a permanent state of partial regression, to reinforce his feelings of helplessness and dependency and to prevent any healthy desire for independent activity. Such permanent pensioners are generally seen by themselves and others as exceedingly unhappy, unfulfilled and blighted men. It has been recommended that any compensation be given in the form of a lump sum only. Some governments, such as that of Canada, have been resistant to the idea of giving pensions to any psychiatric casualties, save those with overt psychosis, Obviously, this is a touchy and explosive area and justice in terms of what is best for the patient may itself become a casualty of interminable wrangling between government officials, the patient and his solicitor.

Another horrifying syndrome, which like the psychiatric disturbances of combat is not unique to the twentieth century but surely is enormously more common during our era than it was before 1914, is the so-called concentration camp syndrome, an ensemble of manifestations resulting from evil, oppressive and coercive social forces of the most damnable type. Many authors, amongst whom Bruno Bettelheim (1960) and Paul Chodoff (1966) are notable, have written hundreds of articles and numerous books on this syndrome. A particularly complete description is provided by Dr Leo Eitinger (1964, 1969), Clinical Director of the Psychiatric Clinic of the University Hospital, University of Oslo, who himself was a prisoner in Auschwitz. His book *Concentration Camp Survivors in Norway and Israel* is a thorough if personal exposition of this entire problem.

The vile story of the concentration camps has been widely publicized in the West and the lessons to be drawn from the story have, we hope, been well learned. The prisoners in Nazi concentration camps and perhaps in concentration camps of other societies whose archives have not come to light were subjected to physical and emotional stresses of unequalled harshness and savagery. They were beaten, injured, tortured, experimented upon, humiliated and worked to an inhuman degree. Each inmate was faced with the threat of imminent death which could occur at any time and for apparently capricious reasons. The prisoners were separated from their families and all basic drives from hunger to sex were perpetually frustrated. Cleanliness was impossible and systematic degradation by brutal guards was the rule. There were certain psychological reactions of an immediate nature to these circumstances. They included regression, shock, terror, outward apathy followed by depression and acute depersonalization. Some individuals appeared to give up and rapidly died. In those who survived longer, such attitudes as irritability, depression, indifference to the sufferings of others, and absorption in the obtaining of food and other advantages were common. Classical psychoneuroses and psychoses were prominently absent: and there is anecdotal evidence to suggest that in the face of such overwhelming reality demands, neurotic behaviour was temporarily extinguished.

It was the hope of the prisoners and of all mankind at the time of liberation that those who had suffered so much would find a happy existence in the post-war world. Unfortunately, this does not seem to have happened. Many of the survivors of the camps have been studied by neurologists and psychiatrists over the intervening quarter of a century, and it is clear that few if any who underwent this cataclysmic experience escaped without scars. There are certain cardinal features of this post-concentration camp syndrome which should be mentioned. All the patients show evidence of persistent underlying anxiety and most of chronic depression. Some of the patients display considerable apathy, dependence, helplessness, and a seclusive and isolationist approach to life. Others are bitter, belligerent, quarrelsome, suspicious and hostile. Psychosomatic disturbances are extremely common, being manifested by gastrointestinal symptoms, fatigue, a sense of exhaustion and of weakness; sleep is invariably disturbed with insomnia, nightmares and restlessness. In addition, there is often the pervasive sense of guilt about the individual's survival at a time when so many people, usually including his relatives, perished in the holocaust. Peter Ostwald and Egon Bittner (1969) have described a sub-group of victims of concentration camps who have developed what the authors call a 'synecdoche of success'. This style of life is characterized by an apparently successful life adjustment based on highly concentrated and aggressive pursuit of success, hiding extreme depression, anxiety and hostility underneath. These victims are outwardly affluent and prosperous but basically unhappy with marked constriction of pleasure, comfort and tranquillity. The authors feel that this phenomenon can be understood in terms of the patients' continuing to perceive the massive threat to existence under which they had always lived as not merely historical but actually as an ever-present reality.

Some authors have attributed many of the persistent psychopathological findings to toxic and traumatic brain lesions resulting from malnutrition, infectious diseases and repeated blows to the head. Other authors emphasize simply the stressful psychic trauma on a scale quite without precedence. In all of human history, even during the Great Inquisition of the past, never was such an effort made systematically and ruthlessly to destroy an entire population, depriving them first of their mental and emotional health and then of their very lives. Certainly there is no other example to be drawn that so clearly illustrates how mental health can be destroyed by malignant and mephitic social forces.

Although war and concentration camps are perhaps the most powerful of social stresses on mental health, there are other major social upheavals which have been associated with psychic disturbances. The influence of social events on such phenomena as suicide is well known. Professor Erwin Stengel, in his splendid volume *Suicide and Attempted Suicide* (1964), has carefully discussed some of these factors. There are many characteristics of individuals correlated with high and low suicide rates. Stengel indicates that 'male sex, increasing age, widowhood, single and divorced state, childlessness, high density of population, residence in big town, high standard of living, economic crises, alcohol consumption, history of a broken home in childhood, mental disorders and physical illness' are associated with high rates of suicide. On the other

Social Factors in the Onset of Disease

hand, such factors as 'female sex, youth, low density of population, rural occupation, religious devoutness, the married state, a large number of children, membership of the lower socio-economic classes, war' are associated with low rates. All of these factors, whether directly or indirectly, relate to the social setting in which people live. There is some evidence, for example, to suggest that in cultures where old age is venerated (rather than despised) such as classical China or some parts of tribal Africa, there is actually a decrease in rates of suicide with increasing age. For another example, the sex differences which were so marked in Western societies at the turn of the century no longer exist so strikingly. During a period of changing roles and statuses for the sexes, the male suicide rate has remained relatively constant, while the female rate has gradually risen so that it now begins to approach the male rate in some areas. Similarly, such factors as residence in a large city or alcoholism are also intimately bound up in the social structure of a given society. The great economic depression which began in the late 1920s and extended until the time of the Second World War was also associated with a rise in suicide rates, whereas the suicide rate during wartime fell. Suicide rates in males are more sensitive to economic cycles than the suicide of females, and economic depression seems to affect the suicide rate of the upper classes more than that of the lower socio-economic groups. Certainly any social forces which increase the losses that an individual might suffer in his accustomed way of life, that is, loss of occupation, status or finances, seems to increase the amount of depressive illness and suicide. Similarly, any attributes of society which weaken the relational system in which people are embedded appears to be associated with increased suicide rate. The suicide rate is highest in the disorganized central sections of cities where schizophrenia is also highest, and it is highest amongst those who have the fewest emotional and social ties to others, namely the single, the widowed, the divorced and the old. So it might be said that in England and America the suicide rate would be the highest for a sixty-year-old white, Protestant, widower living in the centre of a large city such as London or San Francisco, and the lowest rate for a rural, married woman with many children living on a farm in Dorset or South Carolina.

Before we end our discussion on proximal social factors in the onset of mental disease, we should mention work done on migration. Ødegaard (1932) and Malzberg (1962), among others, have found that immigrants to the United States have higher mental hospital admission rates than their former compatriots still living in Europe. Other studies seem to confirm the vulnerability of migrants to mental disease although the differences in rate between migrants and non-migrants are sometimes very slight indeed. On the other hand, still other studies have failed to confirm this notion. Sainsbury (1969) has shown that immigrants to the USA have higher suicide rates (whatever nation they migrate from) than those of their country of origin. Indeed, the suicide rate of immigrant groups is in almost all cases higher than that of the USA as a whole. Similarly the foreign-born display a higher suicide rate in London than do native Englishmen. The question as to whether those who migrate selectively contain individuals who are predisposed to mental illness in greater numbers than in those groups who do not migrate or whether the stress attendant upon leaving one's nation and settling elsewhere in a strange, lonely and alien land is causative of increased mental illness is still an open one. Certainly, a syndrome of 'culture shock' has been widely described in individuals such as Peace Corps men posted overseas for the first time, particularly to areas of non-Western culture. Virtually all these individuals go through some period of depression, irritability and even mild psychosomatic symptoms from which most recover and develop a degree of assimilation. However, there are others who are unable to tolerate this total immersion in an alien culture and who develop a definite psychiatric breakdown not dissimilar to the combat neurosis syndrome. These individuals may have to be evacuated to their homeland.

We have thus seen in this chapter how a series of crises in the life of any individual occurring in rapid succession in a clustering fashion can predispose this individual to the development of an illness, including one of a mental kind. This seems to be particularly true of illnesses of a depressive or psychosomatic nature. We have also seen that monstrous, flagitious, sustained and overwhelming stress, such as occur during combat or incarceration in a concentration camp, can lead to the development of a definite mental syndrome which may be life-long, even in individuals who apparently exhibited neither genetic nor psychological predisposition to such a fate. Similarly, we have seen how such other social forces as economic depressions, migration or the influences of urbanization, secularization, social isolation and anomie can potentiate an increase in a complex emotional phenomenon such as suicide.

6 Transcultural Psychiatry

The accusatory voices heard in the hallucinations of English schizophrenics presumably speak in the English tongue whereas the inner accusations heard by a patient in Madrid are couched in Spanish. This seems to be a trivial enough observation yet it raises many fundamental questions about the nature of psychiatric disease and its relationship to the society in which it occurs. Questions which immediately come to mind include (a) are the mental disease categories found in Western Europe and North America to be found elsewhere in the world? (b) If they are, are the incidence and prevalence of these disorders of the same order of magnitude everywhere, or are there sharp differences in incidence between various societies? (c) Are there particular psychiatric syndromes which are unique to a given society? (d) What are the forces within a given society which seem to affect the incidence, prevalence and types of psychiatric disorder?

Much of the initial data upon which statements in this field have been based are of the impressionistic and non-systematic kind. They consist primarily of observations made by physicians, psychiatrists or others who are more often visitors rather than permanent residents of a given area. A typical observation of this type might be that a certain disorder, let us say, manic-depressive psychosis is rare or common in a certain tribe, region or nation. It is difficult to know what credence can be placed in random statements of this character. At best they can be regarded as clues to the future direction of more extensive and accurate study in the hope that transcultural psychiatry (as Professor Herbert Butterfield wished for history) can be taken out of the hands of 'the strolling minstrels and the pedlars of stories' and accepted 'as a means by which we can gain more understanding of ourselves and our place in the sun'.

Any psychiatric field survey undertaken in locales such as the tropical regions of Africa or Asia must take into account the large number of organic diseases endemic in the native population which may be associated with cerebral manifestations. For example, malaria can give rise to a disturbed mental state which may actually lead to hospitalization in a mental hospital. Similarly, trypanosomiasis or sleeping sickness is commonly associated with various pernicious mental symptoms. Nutritional and vitamin deficiencies, syphilis, and helminthic infestations are also diseases in which there may be associated mental symptoms of a severe type. It is, therefore, necessary to enumerate carefully such cases and separate them from those cases which appear to represent a 'pure' mental disease, perhaps more accurately called a functional mental disorder of presently unknown etiology. Another complication in comparing rates and varieties of mental illness in different cultures and different nations comes about because of different training of physicians who do the diagnosing. Pierre Pichot (1967), of the Faculty of Medicine at Paris, has shown how American, English-speaking psychiatrists differ from French psychiatrists in their use of concepts of mental illness, and even in the use of words that are spelled similarly in the two languages, but have decidedly different connotations.

There is a growing volume of papers reported in such publications as the *British Journal of Psychiatry* or the *Trans-Cultural Psychiatric Research Review and Newsletter* which deal with transcultural findings. They add up to a body of literature of the most variegated and heterogeneous kind describing such topics as suicide in Hong Kong, depression in Burma, obsessive compulsive neurosis in Nyasaland, and so forth. It is extraordinarily difficult to draw general conclusions from so varied a mass of material. Instead, at this point, it might be helpful to discuss certain major illustrative studies in the field of transcultural psychiatry (also called cross-cultural psychiatry or ethnopsychiatry or occasionally psychiatric anthropology).

Some years ago, between 1946 and 1948, Dr T. Y. Lin (1953) of the World Health Organization carried out his first epidemiological study of psychiatric disorders on the island of Taiwan (Formosa). Fifteen years later Lin (1966) carried out a similar epidemiological survey. He studied all Taiwanese who were of Chinese descent living in three sample districts: a rural district of five villages; a small town; and a section of a large city. Approximately 20,000 people were studied in three stages. In the first stage the research team visited all the leaders of the community, for example, the mayor, the district or village chief, census and welfare officials, elders, health workers, schoolmasters and police. Information was obtained from updated census registers and police records as well as from the various informants. Data were obtained on the size of each family and the age, sex, education, occupation and social class of various members. In the second stage of investigation, which lasted about two to three months (the first stage having run about four to six months), detailed psychiatric information was obtained on all cases reported in the first stage of the investigation. In addition, further psychiatric cases were sought out through the use of hospital and clinic records. In the final stage of the survey, a psychiatric team visited every inhabitant of the district. Anyone who was felt to be mentally ill was then referred to the principal investigator, Lin, for his personal examination and final certification as a case. Fifteen years later, essentially the same study was carried out again in the same areas. Fortunately the research team remained stable so that comparable approaches and criteria were used each time. Obviously the years between 1946 and 1961 were extremely eventful years for Formosa with marked changes in population, economic status and culture. At the time of the first study a prevalence rate of 10·8 per 1000 population for diagnosable mental disorder was obtained. There was also litttle variation in rate between the three types of communities. The type of disorders seen and their prevalence were considered to be within the same order of magnitude as exists in Western Europe and the United States. Previously there had been speculations that Chinese society might be free of mental disorder.

Certainly, if this Formosan sample is any indication, that conjecture is not true. Fifteen years later the prevalence rate had risen to 16·9 per 1000 population, a significantly higher figure. As expected, the prevalence rates for psychoses had not changed. The rise was accounted for primarily by higher rates of psychoneuroses, psychopathic personality disorders and mental deficiency. It was suggested that the enormous social and economic changes in Formosa following the end of the Chinese Civil War played some role in the change in prevalence figures.

Another careful field study is that of Leighton, Lambo and many others of the Cornell Program in Social Psychiatry (1963), who studied the Yoruba people of Nigeria in the early 1960s. Their approach to the Yoruba study employed many of the same approaches used in the Stirling County Study in Nova Scotia. The major findings from this field survey was that, although there were some significant differences in the differential prevalence of various subtypes of mental disorders between Nigeria and Nova Scotia, the 'similarity in the two samples is much more impressive than the differences'. Differences included such things as a greater level of psychophysiological complaints amongst the Yoruba than in Nova Scotia. However, there was a higher prevalence of organic disease in the Yoruba so that such complaints as headache, respiratory difficulties, skin trouble, genito-urinary complaints might very well have been connected with nutritional, parasitic or infectious disease rather than being psychogenic. There was also a greater level of psychoneurotic symptoms in the Nigerian sample than in Stirling County. Psychotic individuals were uncommon in both samples but those seen fell into recognizable diagnostic categories such as schizophrenia. On the other hand, drug addiction was not found at all amongst the Yoruba.

One further example of an important field study on a selected population is the study of Joseph W. Eaton and Robert J. Weil (1955) on mental health in the Hutterite Communities of the North American Middle West, reported in their book *Culture and Mental Disorders*. The Hutterites are a fundamentalist religious sect who live in strict isolation in a section of the Middle West of North America, particularly in the States of North and South Dakota, Montana and in the prairie provinces of Canada. They are an extremely cohesive and closely knit group of German descent who lived in Russia and then migrated to the United States in the 1870s. They dwell in ninety-eight colonies in which simple living, communal ownership of property, and passivism predominate, and renunciation of worldly pleasures such as radio and the cinema is universal. They are all literate and are expert in efficient and specialized agriculture. Prior to the authors' study it was said that mental disorders were essentially unknown amongst the Hutterites. They never appeared as patients in mental hospitals and physicians thought that they showed few psychiatric symptoms. In fact, the provincial legislature of Manitoba was told in 1947 that there was 'a complete absence of mental illness' in the Hutterite colonies. This idyllic picture did not stand up to close scrutiny. 8542 Hutterites were screened by the research team and a total of 199 individuals were found who either had active symptoms of a mental disorder or who had recovered from one. Fifty-three of these illnesses were diagnosed as psychosis. Therefore, the total overall prevalence rate approximated that of other field surveys in urban areas showing that the Hutterite culture provided no certain defence against the outbreak of mental disorders of certain types. However, the distribution of mental illnesses was markedly different from that of other areas in the United States and Canada. For example, there was no evidence of any kind of anti-social behaviour. None of the patients had histories of murder, sexual perversion, assault, arson or even marital break-up. Similarly, there was no evidence of alcoholism, drug addiction or syphilis. On the other hand depressive illnesses were extraordinarily common and psychotic depressions outnumbered cases of schizophrenia, a reversal of the usual ratio. Prominent in the symptom picture shown by neurotic Hutterites were depressive feelings, remorse, guilt, self-blame and vague psychosomatic disorders such as headaches, backaches, hysterical paralyses, and so forth. The authors were struck by the wide range of personality types and individual differences they encountered even in a society which stressed continuous indoctrination, identical clothing, cooking and life schedules.

These three studies were chosen as being illustrative ones and also because they employed careful case finding techniques in an attempt to establish true prevalence rates. Had Eaton and Weil relied on mental hospital statistics for their information they would have found no Hutterite cases at all since mentally ill Hutterites were only sent to the hospital under the most extreme circumstances and then for only short periods in order to receive electro-shock therapy. Obviously then, reports from distant places utilizing mental hospital data only are to be considered with great caution because the hospitalized patients may represent a very select and skewed sample of the mentally ill in a given community. The random and undocumented observations of travellers or general physicians or even psychiatrists resident in a given area must be regarded with similar suspicion.

If these three studies can be considered accurate and representative, it would appear that mental disease is a feature of human society throughout the globe. We already know that mental illness is highly prevalent in Western Europe and North America, at least in the urban areas. Apparently agricultural societies of a traditional sort are not free from mental disease either. Similarly, many of the major types of mental illness common in the West, for example, schizophrenia, manic-depressive psychosis and psychoneurosis were also noted in Asia and African populations. However, while certain core symptoms were present of sufficient magnitude to make the cases diagnosable by psychiatrists, the clinical manifestations were clearly influenced in some measure by the social forces of a given society from which the patients sprang.

Murphy, Wittkower and Chance (1964) conducted a cross-cultural inquiry into the symptomatology of depression. A questionnaire was completed by psychiatrists from thirty different nations in Africa, Asia, Australasia, the Middle East, Europe, North America and Latin America. In all cases, the respondents reported that they saw patients who displayed a depressive syndrome defined by 'a mood of depression or dejection: diurnal mood change; insomnia with early morning wakening; diminution of interest in social environment'. They further found that fatigue, loss of sexual interest, self-accusatory ideas, anorexia and weight loss were frequently associated with the 'core syndrome of depressive states'. However, such symptoms as guilt and self-depreciation tended to occur only in patients of Western Christian cultural background and were largely absent in patients from other cultures.

Another study which clearly indicates the influence of cultural patterns on the expression of symptoms in patients with a given mental disease is the study of Italian-American and Irish-American schizophrenics in New York City by Marvin K. Opler (1959). Opler studied seventy-seven hospitalized male schizophrenics, forty Irish and thirty-seven Italian. In each case the diagnosis was thought to be unequivocal and most had received extensive hospitalization and treatment including electro-shock treatments. Opler was able to show, however, that the patients differed strikingly in the expression of certain characteristics. For example, it was postulated that because schizophrenics are 'notoriously troubled by homosexual strivings' these patients would also show difficulties in this area but the expression of the difficulties would be determined by cultural factors. It was thought that the Italians (who were all from the south of Italy) would display their struggles more openly and actively than the Irish, who were thought to be particularly prone to the repression of sexual expression of any kind. This was found to be the case, with the Italian patients showing poorly controlled sexual impulses and direct expression of sexuality without apparent preoccupation with guilt and with the thoughts of having sinned because of the mere possession of sexual impulses. The groups differed in many other dimensions. For example, alcoholism was more common among the Irish than in the Italian-American patients. Hypochondriasis, fixed delusional systems and a complaint attitude towards authority were also more common in the Irish than in the Italian group. This differential prevalence of symptoms was traced to the psychosocial patterns inherent in the differing family structures and family interactions in the two subcultures. The Italian culture was seen to emphasize emotional expression and overt action. Italian schizophrenic patients would thus tend to express their problems in overt behavioural terms. The Irish culture was seen to act to inhibit sexuality, to emphasize male inadequacy, fear of females and latent homosexual tendencies. The inculcation of a sense of sin and guilt was seen to have exaggerated expression in schizophrenic patients with their weak and fragmented egos. It is as if these extremely disturbed and disorganized patients show in the most exaggerated and characteristic way all the conflicts, demands and imperatives of the society which are thrown into sharp relief by the extraordinary yet thought-provoking speech and behaviour of the psychotic patients.

It would be quite amazing if psychiatric disease occurred with the same frequency in all societies. This uniformity would be absolutely contrary to the distribution of virtually every other biological or social phenomenon in human life. Certainly, organic diseases are not evenly distributed over the globe, and nations indeed differ in their customs and cultural patterns. The uniformity of mental disease patterns found in various surveys is perhaps more surprising than the differences, considering the varying genetic and environmental aspects of life in Midtown Manhattan as compared to life in Western Nigeria or rural Formosa. Human existence does have some common threads which unite all mankind. Work, marriage, play, stress and death know no societal boundaries. Unfortunately, psychiatric epidemiology is still in the exploratory stage of documenting differences rather than being able to move on to exploring the reasons why these differences exist. Speculations are common enough in this area but one wishes for more solid evidence to back up what often seem to be rather thin conjectures.

One body of work currently in progress which promises to document carefully the differences in the prevalence of psychopathology in two areas is the Bilateral Project on Diagnosis of Mental Disorders in the US and UK. It was previously mentioned in chapter 3 that there were striking differences in the admission rate for certain disorders, particularly manic-depressive psychosis, between the United States and the United Kingdom. Various investigators have been involved in developing instruments carefully standardized for use in both areas. In addition, they have been working on developing laboratory tests and in examining the processes by which the clinicians in each nation arrive at a final diagnosis. The advantages of studying these two nations in so careful a fashion have been pointed out by Kendell (1969). There are in the United States and the United Kingdom well developed and extensive psychiatric facilities and physicians trained in psychiatry for a comparable length of time in similar programmes of training. There is, in addition, a common language and reasonably careful records are kept. However, it would appear from the information already developed in this study that there are differences in diagnostic styles between American and British psychiatrists, with American psychiatrists tending to use the diagnosis of schizophrenia more often than the British do. This notion was tested by means of such procedures as structured psychiatric interviews made independently by various members of a team and by the use of video tapes on selected patients, tapes being exchanged back and forth across the Atlantic. It also appears that in addition to any inclination for American psychiatrists to diagnose psychotic patients as schizophrenic and for English psychiatrists to see them as manic-depressive, there appears to be a genuine difference in the prevalence of manic-depressive disorders between the two countries. At present, this disease would appear to be genuinely more common in the United Kingdom than it is in the United States.

Another revealing study indicating striking differences between two cultural groups in terms of their types of psychiatric disorders is that of the Filipinos in the US Navy. Duff and Arthur (1966) described the psychiatric problems of sailors who are citizens of the Philippine Republic but who enlist in the US Navy for active service. These men are all carefully selected and are of a similar age and level of education to American recruits. They also pass a very rigorous physical examination before entering the service. Since there are many more candidates than there are places, those chosen have met a high standard. The attrition rate of cohorts of Filipino recruits is far less than that of their American counterparts and in all periods through their naval career they show a smaller rate of premature discharge from the service than do their American contemporaries. The Filipino rate of admission to the psychiatric sick list is also far below the general naval level; however, when one examines Filipino psychiatric admissions, one is struck not only by their relative scarcity but by their extreme diagnostic homogeneity. Psychoneuroses, organic brain syndromes, character and behaviour disorders are conspicuous by their absence. Instead, about three-quarters of the cases fall into a diagnostic category of paranoid schizophrenia. The clinical picture that is seen proves to be a very stereotyped one characterized by suspiciousness, ideas of reference, bizarre and disordered thinking, often delusions of persecution and invariably a severe and protracted hypochondriasis marked by peculiar pains felt everywhere in the body. While there is surprising uniformity of agreement among naval physicians seeing these patients in the scattered units of the fleet as to the diagnosis of paranoid schizophrenia, the patients themselves see their symptoms in quite another light. They dwell upon their somatic symptoms such as pain and consider them part of a syndrome called Pasma Sa Ugat which is common in the Philippine Islands and which, in their view, is best treated by a native practitioner utilizing certain traditional and, to those educated in the western medical tradition, magical procedures. There are no objective data available as to the adequacy of the native therapists, indeed, this lack of information characterizes all discussions about native practitioners. However, it is clearly true that the patients seldom seem to show any marked improvement following treatment in naval hospitals and most have to be returned to the Philippine Islands for further treatment. Incidently, a major civilian mental hospital in the Philippines also reported a preponderance of psychotic cases of the paranoid schizophrenic type in their patient population.

It was postulated by the authors that certain features of the culture of the Philippine Islands, particularly child-rearing practices which emphasize passivity and the discouragement of outward expressions of aggression, play a role in the development of the particular symptom picture, although perhaps not at all in the basic etiology of the disorder itself.

There is one type of medical problem certainly involving the mind, the emotions, the body as well as society, which shows extreme differences of prevalence and form in various societies. This is the problem of alcoholism. In their book *Alcoholism and Society*, Chafetz and Demone (1962) have extensively discussed the interaction between drinking habits, alcoholic addiction and social pressures. Alcohol has been available to virtually all human societies for millenniums, yet there are societies both primitive and advanced with very low rates of compulsive addiction to alcohol. On the other hand, some societies or some social groups within societies in advanced nations or in nations undergoing rapid social change, show a high rate of alcoholism. In most preliterate groups such as Aleut Indians and the Indians of the Andes drinking occurs in carefully prescribed social situations. These are usually group drinking activities where there may be considerable release of tension and outwardly wild behaviour but always within the pattern set forth by the group. Alcohol is used as a means of enhancement of social relationships and social pleasure rather than as some form of compulsively consumed anodyne. In addition, there are no feelings of ambivalence or sinfulness involved in the drinking process.

In western societies the Jews and Italians have very low rates of alcoholism. In these two cultural groups alcohol consumption is an integral part of socialization and of group rites rather than being individual and sporadic. On the other hand, in America, the Irish-American ethnic group has always had a rate of alcoholism many times that of any other group. It is postulated that historical and social factors in Irish society, which have encouraged high rates of alcohol consumption, particularly in men, when added to the deprivations found in the American environment all combined to produce a societal group in which alcoholism would be common.

There have been described over the years a number of unique syndromes specific to a time and place. These are sometimes called 'exotic' psychiatric syndromes. An exotic area, of course, is generally conceived of as being some place far enough away to be unknown. Thus, Kansas City is exotic to a Singaporian but not to a Kansan, and Darjeeling seems very exotic from the perspective of Bournemouth but scarcely so to a Darjeeling man.

One culture-specific aberrant mental state or 'exotic' psychiatric syndrome occurring in Malaya, North Africa and Northern Asia is termed latah. Patients with this disorder are usually middle-aged or elderly females who, following a supposedly sudden traumatic experience of some type, develop a state similar to that of hypnotic suggestability and imitate directly what other people say and do. This is known as echolalia and echopraxia. The patient may imitate animals or other objects in nature. In addition, the patient may mumble obscenities or make frankly sexual gestures. Some of the patients may develop a full blown chronic psychosis, in other cases they may have merely paroxysms of latah lasting for some months. The individuals affected by this disorder appear to be people who are very passive, of rather low intelligence and, in general, obsequious and compliant even before the latah appeared. It would seem as if the person exhibiting this syndrome has surrendered her will entirely to others and has abdicated all aggressivity and responsibility in this surrender.

Another syndrome which used to be well known in the South-East Asia area, particularly in the Philippines, Indonesia and Malaya, is known as amok. This syndrome occurs in males of a retiring disposition. These individuals appear first to go into a characteristic depressive withdrawal featured by what appears to be intense brooding silence. Suddenly the person with amok cries out, seizes a weapon and proceeds on a headlong beserk charge, killing everything in his path. The usual fate of the amok male is either to be killed or to kill himself, after he has injured or murdered a number of other people and/or even animals. A similar type of behaviour known as 'wild man' is said to occur in the highlands of New Guinea.

During recent years when shifts in cultural values have occurred amok has declined in incidence. Amok might be regarded as an outburst of massive rage in a basically schizoid and depressed person channelled by cultural sanctions into a particular syndrome. As the values of the culture have changed under the influences of the modern world the sanctions formerly given to outbursts like amok have disappeared, and the syndrome has correspondingly declined in incidence. Homicide and suicide still continue to occur in these societies, as a glance at the pages of recent history will attest; however, they no longer tend to occur in this highly ritualistic and stylized form.

Another syndrome involving a stereotyped kind of wild behaviour occurs among the Polar Eskimo, and is known as pibloktoq. This syndrome is characterized by frenzy, coprophagia, tearing off one's clothing, imitating animals, and so forth. Following the seizure, the victims, as is the case with the victims of latah or the few survivors of amok, claim amnesia for the episode.

Another peculiar syndrome of Eskimos of the Hudson Bay area and of the Ogibwa Indians of south-east Ontario is known as whitico or windigo. This syndrome is also characterized by brooding withdrawal and, at least historically, by attacks on relatives and cannibalism. Its name comes from the fancied resemblance of the syndrome to a spirit figure known as a whitico which is an ice skeleton that practises cannibalism.

Other types of cultural specific syndromes primarily involving sexual conflicts rather than aggressive ones are the Ufufuyana syndrome seen in the Bantu of South Africa and the koro syndrome seen in the Southern Chinese. In the Ufufuyana syndrome, women develop hysterical paralyses, pains, seizures and nightmares about being assaulted by a dwarf-like spirit figure well known in the culture.

In koro, which also occurs in the Celebese and in West Borneo as well as in South China, a male begins to fear that his penis is disappearing into his abdomen and when it finally does he will die. During the attack the victim employs various means to prevent this from occurring, including holding the penis, having relatives hold it, or fastening it with some kind of a wooden clasp to prevent its withdrawal. The explanation given in the culture is that there is an overabundance of female principle or 'yin' in the individual that is causing the penile withdrawal. This excess yin must be counteracted by administration of some medicines which contain the male principle or yang.

There are numerous other syndromes such as voodoo death, voodoo trances or spirit possession reported from around the world. In each of these cases it would seem as if individuals who are suffering from some primary sort of mental illness, perhaps schizophrenia, perhaps organic brain syndrome, or perhaps hysteria, have their feelings of deep anxiety about aggression and sex, those universal concerns, channelled into a prescribed symptom pattern which is powerfully sanctioned within the culture.

Individuals in primitive cultures are treated by a wide variety of healing practices; however, basic to all the treatment methods are a series of culturally accepted explanations as to the causation of the disease phenomena, faith in the healer, and certain ritualistic practices on his part which are often designed to deal with unconscious conflicts and to use group values to strengthen the individual's desire to return to the society. Data are simply not available as to the efficacy of these methods even if it were clear as to what criteria would be used to judge results.

As one looks at psychiatric disease around the world in preliterate societies, developing nations and in technologically advanced nations there are some similarities to be seen. In the first place, whenever a given group or society is studied carefully mental illnesses are found within the population. In the second place, there appear to be inter-group variations in the prevalences of the different psychiatric disorders.

I would venture to suggest on the basis of the present evidence that the disorders range along a continuum with psychoses on one end and phenomena such as juvenile delinquency and perhaps alcoholism on the other. In the case of the major psychoses the core symptoms are readily apparent in the patients of any culture; however, the degree and type of various other manifestations are obviously bound up with the particular cultural background of the individual afflicted. On the other end of the continuum, there are societies, such as the Hutterites, where the social pressures are such that drug addiction, alcoholism and juvenile delinquency do not appear. Clearly, as Leighton and Hughes (1961) point out, the culture, through its child-rearing practices, sanctions, taboos and other indoctrination procedures, encourages certain traits and discourages others. These traits may appear in exaggerated or pathological form in the mental illnesses which afflicted members of the society develop. A culture may also produce vulnerable personality types and give prestige to certain manifestations, such as hallucinations or hysterical seizures, which in other cultures would be regarded as psycho-pathological. Finally, a society might predispose itself so the development of certain psychiatric disorders by its physical mode of living, e.g. preferentially living in an area where cerebral malaria or insect-borne encephalitis is common. A society might conceivably, through selective breeding practices, say, father–daughter incest, make itself vulnerable to the development of a high incidence of those mental disorders which appear to be inherited. In the area of mental disorders there is indeed a panoply of potential outcomes in the interaction of culture, individual traits and inherited constitution.

7 Social Psychiatry in the Hospital Setting

Hospitals were not always the gleaming cities of hope that they may occasionally appear to be today. Past generations in the Western world and present generations in other areas of the earth have rightly regarded the hospital with suspicion and foreboding, as a place where many entered but few left cured. Indeed we now know that many hospitals of past centuries were really anti-therapeutic in the sense that they provided superb concentration points for pathogenic bacteria as well as being the venue for some remarkably unphysiological medical practices such as blood letting, a procedure which must have hastened the demise of many a patient. Today, of course, one learns of outbreaks of infectious disease even in the most advanced hospitals and of patients who suffer from the toxic effects of modern therapy. On the whole, however, people expect (with a certain degree of accuracy) to receive in hospital good and at times spectacular treatment for all manner of bodily ills.

What has been true of the bad past reputation of the general hospital has been *a fortiori* true of the mental hospital. The prototype hospital which comes to mind is that of Bedlam (the Hospital of St Mary of Bethlehem in London). No one would have imagined that therapeutic good ever came from such a place. Its only apparent beneficent effect was the protection of the general public from supposedly dangerous lunatics. As previously mentioned, in the early nineteenth century, some mental hospitals of the York Retreat type became model institutions which appeared to do good for those patients who came there seeking help, at least as far as we can infer from the statistics available. After this brief and apparently false dawn, mental hospitals once again became institutions of diminished reputation. However, they seemed to exist almost out of public consciousness until well into the twentieth century.

In this century psychiatric hospitals at various times have received the full candle power of newspaper and magazine publicity. The inhuman and shameful conditions of many state mental hospitals in the United States (and some of their counterparts abroad) were glaringly revealed by enterprising journalists. At a more academic level, sociologists, social psychologists and social psychiatrists discovered the possibilities of studying the mental hospital as a social institution. Over the last several decades a flood of books and journal articles on the social aspects of mental hospitals has appeared. Both journalists and sociologists seemed to have agreed that many if not most features of life in a large mental hospital have been actually harmful to the health of the patients brought there for treatment. However, there is a difference in emphasis between the two sets of accounts. The journalistic descriptions stressed the overcrowding, the rampant physical disease such as amoebic dysentery and tuberculosis, the poor food which leads to malnutrition and hypovitaminosis, and the low ratio of staff to patients which resulted in extremely limited and depersonalized care. The popular accounts have often also described some psychopathological tendencies amongst the staff who were confronted with so overwhelming a burden of patient care. On the other hand such accounts almost always mentioned extremely selfless and dedicated workers who have devoted their entire lives to patient care in an unglamourous and frequently traduced environment.

In contrast to the journalists, the sociologists have been primarily interested in the social structure, organizational aspects, ideology, social roles and interpersonal interactions of the hospital and its staff. These workers, as well as many psychiatrists and psychologists, have postulated, for example, that certain ideological and organizational aspects of the mental hospital structure have worked to the detriment of patients. The main idea is that the patient entering the mental hospital, most commonly a patient with schizophrenia, has certain deficits characteristic of the disease itself such as disturbances in the thinking process, bizarre emotional responsivity, delusional ideas and perhaps hallucinations. It is further postulated that in the old custodial type hospital with its sterile, monotonous and frequently repressive atmosphere, the patient developed a whole new set of symptoms and other handicaps derived from environmental pressures which were then engrafted onto the basic disease process. These implants and elaborations might include stereotyped mannerisms and regressive behaviour such as soiling, coprophragia, self-mutilation and so forth. Wing (1967) distinguished between these two phenomena by calling them primary and secondary handicaps in schizophrenia. It is to the prevention of the secondary handicap that much of the work in hospital social psychiatry and related community psychiatry has addressed itself.

There are several important works which are both illustrative and representative of the large body of literature on the social aspects of mental hospitals. In 1954, Stanton and Schwartz (1954) published their pioneering work, *The Mental Hospital*. The authors, who were by profession a psychiatrist and a sociologist respectively, studied a small private mental hospital specializing in the treatment of psychoses by intensive psychotherapy. They viewed the hospital as an integrated social system imbedded in which were various social subsystems which had to function at an adequate level in order to fulfill the purposes of the hospital. They showed how various interactional processes and institutional patterns had effects on both the behaviour and the therapeutic course of the patients and they identified specific ways in which these staff interactions affected the patients.

Within the structure of the mental hospital is a system of roles assigned to various staff members. A mental hospital is organized along hierarchical lines, for example, doctor, nurse, ward attendant, with mobility between statuses completely blocked. If an individual wishes to change status from that of ward attendant to nurse or from nurse to physician, he or she would have to leave the institution to take further training elsewhere in order to accomplish this promotion. However, there was in the actual operation of the hospital a good deal of confusion about specific aspects of patient care responsibility characterized by a lack of clear definition of the several staff roles, overlapping roles and ambiguity in the minds of the staff as to what their precise responsibilities were. Such role confusion within the staff, in the experience of Stanton and Schwartz, inevitably resulted in corresponding confusion amongst the patients. The authors reported how a disagreement about the handling of a case between such individuals as the physician directly in charge of the case and his administrative supervisor or between the ward nurse and the supervising physician could be shown to cause increasing disturbance and regression in the patient. They felt that the patient's disturbance was all the greater if the disagreement, although quite real, remained covert and was not brought out into the open to be aired, discussed and, one might hope, settled. Underlying the staff disagreements, quite apart from either the so-called medical facts of the case or even personal animosity amongst staff members unconnected with their work, were such difficulties as faulty communication between staff members and between patients and staff. There might be inaccurate, misleading and false information passed or information with many omissions or gross distortions. During the times when there was blockage of free and accurate communication between patients and staff, the patients might then develop their own separate social structure and communications network. In addition to role ambiguities and defective communication channels another area of importance in the production of adverse reactions amongst the hospitalized patients was faulty decision making. Stanton and Schwartz studied the structure and dynamics of decision making and the general exercise of power in the mental hospital. As might be expected, on occasions when it was not clear as to who was making the decision about some aspect of ward policy or where there was no opportunity for lower level staff members to have any part in the decisions, there was some impairment of performance on the part of the staff which in turn resulted in patient disturbance. During the staff disagreements there appeared to be little interchange of actual cognitive information but a good deal of covert emotional interchange which the authors dubbed a 'split social field'. They felt that such 'split social fields' were productive of a good deal of patient and staff anxiety as well as excitement and sudden outbreaks amongst the patients of rage, crying or other overt emotional displays.

Their work had a powerful impact on psychiatric thinking not so much because of the novelty of their views, since many similar ideas had been written and talked about for years, but rather because they were able to bring these notions together and place them in a coherent framework. By utilizing one small hospital they were able to show in a quite convincing fashion how the entire social structure of the hospital and the personal interactions of its staff affected the clinical course of the patients.

Although quite different in character from the work of Stanton and Schwartz, *Asylums* by Erving Goffman (1961) is also seminal. The book is in the form of several extended essays rather than being a report of scientific investigations, but while its literary character detracts from its scientific definitiveness the book more than makes up for that loss by its power and impact.

Professor Goffman begins by defining the characteristics of what he calls 'total institutions' into which category he places homes for the blind, the aged, orphans and the indigent, tuberculosis sanitoria, mental hospitals, leprosaria, penitentiaries, prisoner-of-war camps, concentration camps, army barracks, ships, boarding schools, work camps, colonial compounds, large mansions, abbeys, monasteries, convents and other cloisters. These institutions are held to break down the barriers between sleep, play and work, which normally obtain in modern Western civilization. Characteristically, there is a single plan for the fulfilment of the official objectives of such institutions. In order to accomplish this plan, life for the inmates has to be conducted under a single authority in the same place, in the immediate company of others, and under a tight and explicitly formulated schedule. In total institutions there is a basic split between a managed group whom he calls 'inmates' and a smaller 'staff' whose major function is 'surveillance – a seeing to it that everyone does what he has been clearly told is required of him, under conditions where one person's infraction is likely to stand out in relief against the visible, constantly examined compliance of the others'. Goffman regards the differentiation of staff and inmates as basic, with a vast social distance intervening between them. Each group is supposed to view the other in pejorative terms, that is, the staff views the inmates as 'bitter, secretive and untrustworthy' whilst inmates view the staff as 'condescending, high-handed and mean'. The world of the inmate is seen as one in which identity must be surrendered, self-mortified, and autonomy and freedom of action lost. In addition, the inmate must learn about the so-called 'privilege system', a series of formal and informal rules by which he must live in order to get along in the institution. These rules are primarily concerned with obedience to the staff and transgressions are invariably punished. For example, on a hospital ward the attendant can give favourite patients better jobs, better beds, certain amenities such as coffee or tea, increased privacy or even increased freedom to move about the grounds. On the other hand, the attendant, even without reference to the physician in charge, can punish by such means as sarcasm, ridicule, taking away of privileges and so forth. In his essay, 'The underlife of a public institution: A study of ways of making out in a mental hospital' (1961), appearing in the same volume, Goffman describes in rich and exquisite detail all the ways in which the system attempts to influence control and indoctrinate the patients. He also delineates even more ingenious ways by which the patients attempt to avoid the system in the areas of territoriality, personal possessions, brief interludes of privacy, reading, personal contacts, personal grooming, and so forth. The life of the patients during the twenty-three or more hours a day that they are not in contact with the psychiatrists is vividly portrayed. Even in hospital only a favourite few patients see the doctor as much as an hour a day and some patients in large mental hospitals are fortunate if they see the doctor for a total of an hour in six months.

The patient lives within the medical environment of the

hospital and is also embedded in the underlife of the mental institution. In this setting the patients experiences a 'moral career'. This term is used to mean the enormous social and institutional pressures placed upon the patient forcing him towards the adoption of a relatively stereotyped role as a 'sick patient' who is willingly accepting medical treatment for his condition. This indoctrination is presumed to begin in the pre-patient period when the shaping is done by relatives and corrosive social forces such as the police or judges. Once within the hospital the whole weight of the total institution including the system of segregating patients by wards and the ideological conviction of the entire staff act as a powerful force of indoctrination. The clinical records, staff conferences, group sessions, and so forth are utilized piteously to reveal all the secrets which the patients might wish to conceal and to remorselessly build up an airtight case proving that the patient is indeed mentally sick, has behaved shamefully and that in order to be restored to the society of ordinary men he must place himself entirely in the staff's hands and follow out their programme of indoctrination and instruction, called medical treatment.

Goffman later goes on, naturally enough, to point out the deficiencies inherent in the utilization of a medical model for the operation of a mental hospital. As was alluded to in earlier chapters, the entire rationale for the construction and operation of mental hospitals is that mental illnesses are diseases, albeit of a peculiar type, and that the problems raised by mental illness in society are best handled by treating the possessors of these illnesses as if they were medical patients, utilizing a medical service model in their treatment and rehabilitation. If one does not accept this basic premise, of course, then one must abjure the entire notion of the structure and functioning of such hospitals.

Goffman does not accept the premise and thus attacks the whole idea of mental hospitals although he admits that hospitals are useful to some of the individuals who are institutionalized as 'patients'. He also indicates that he has no suggestion at this time of any better way of handling mental patients. The hospitals were, after all, built as a presumed response to a given problem rather than as institutions to provide employment. He ends by saying:

> Mental patients can find themselves in a special bind. To get out of the hospital, or to ease their life within it, they must show acceptance of the place accorded them, and the place accorded them is to support the occupational role of those who appear to force this bargain. This self-alienating moral servitude, which perhaps helps to account for some inmates becoming mentally confused, is achieved by invoking the great tradition of the expert servicing relation, especially its medical variety. Mental patients can find themselves crushed by the weight of a service deal that eases life for the rest of us.

There is no doubt that Professor Goffman has provided us with a fascinatingly written and highly discerning picture of life in the total institution, particularly a mental hospital, as seen from the standpoint of the patient. On the other hand, one must regard the work as tendentious in character. In the first place there is certainly some doubt that the institutions are quite as total, quite as monolithic, and the staff quite as omnipotent as one might suppose from reading this work. There are indeed poor souls who succumb totally to indoctrination wherever given, whether it be in a Chinese commune or a mental hospital, but one tends to be impressed rather with the enormous amount of mental reservations, obduracy, and stubborn obstructionism which so many people possess. This implacable individualism has been a source of discomfort to tyrants throughout the ages and obstructs those on a mental hospital staff who harbour tyrannical wishes. Karmel (1969) has shown that self-mortification as well as loss of self-esteem and social identity did not occur amongst patients studied in a 'total institution' (a New York State mental hospital). She suggests that what appears to an outsider to be humiliating, mortifying and 'role-dispossessing' in mental hospital treatment may not appear as such to the patient who may regard many of the treatment measures taken as helpful rather than distressing.

Furthermore, individuals who have mental illnesses which are mediated through defective functioning of the brain and who are receiving powerful drugs undoubtedly profit from being under close supervision to monitor their clinical course and to watch for signs of serious or possibly fatal drug toxicity.

There probably is also a need for society and its various subunits such as the family to sequester, at least temporarily, certain individuals whose behaviour and thinking is grossly disordered and disruptive. Obviously, some might argue that this should never be done involuntarily and that relatives and society should treat at home all individuals no matter how disordered their conduct. On the other hand, there is certainly a strong body of opinion to show that certain individuals with mental illness are genuine threats to themselves or to others and not merely social troublemakers whom tyrannical judges, compliant prosecutors and wicked doctors wish to imprison. For example, there are some patients who, in the course of acute manic psychosis, systematically destroy their economic, occupational and family life. There are others who, in the course of depression, pose a real danger of suicide. There are patients with acute schizophrenia who pose an equal danger of homicide. Hospitalization may be regarded as a boon for such unfortunates. There is also some evidence to show that the continued presence of a severely mentally ill patient within the family has deleterious effects on the psychological functioning of children in the home.

However, if present trends of decreasing hospital patient populations continue, the entire question of the alleged deleterious impact of the mental hospital on the patients' dignity and clinical course may become an academic or an historical one. Certainly, if present figures are extrapolated into the future decades this final emptying of the mental hospitals will come about before the end of the century. However, it is never warranted to assume that present trends must necessarily continue. It might well be that the curves of declining resident patients in mental hospitals may show a levelling off in the future and there will remain in hospital a residual group of patients who are unable to be discharged in spite of all possible therapeutic measures. If this phenomenon does indeed occur explanations for it would differ. Those medically inclined would indicate that there is a group of patients with sufficient disturbance of brain and mental function as to preclude their operating successfully in the ordinary world. Those favouring the conspiratorial approach might argue this patient group would be a residual one composed of the greatest troublemakers or the most burdensome to society who are to be left in medical concentration camps to keep them out of society's way.

It should be clearly recognized that there are, in fact, at least two major streams of criticism of the mental hospital. The first, which accepts the inevitability of some kind of psychiatric hospital or service, even if part of a general hospital, has focused on the deplorable conditions in many mental hospitals. Critics of this type have railed against the vast overcrowding, the endemic diseases, the poor and monotonous diet, the horrid quarters, the exiguous treatment resources and, most notably, the paucity of trained staff to carry out psychotherapeutic regimens. This group would accept mental hospitals as potentially good if only they were well equipped and fully staffed.

The other group, of which Goffman might stand as a notably eloquent example, would argue that the increased staffing, rather than being a good might, in fact, be an evil because with increased group sessions, individual psychotherapy, and so forth, the pressures for indoctrination of the patient into accepting the concept that he is mentally ill, that he has transgressed the mores of the society and that he can only be cured by confession and reconstitution would be even more immense than they are at present. Currently, of course, in many hospitals the staff size is so small that many patients have rather little opportunity or necessity, if you will, to reveal at length their secret problems and feelings.

Over the past few decades there have been many humane psychiatrists who, while dissatisfied with what they regarded as a custodial outlook on the part of the staffs of mental hospitals and other psychiatric centres, have been unwilling to renounce the therapeutic potential inherent in the general social context of such institutions. A good example of the use of social forces in a residential hospital setting for the treatment of individuals with deviant behaviour is the 'therapeutic community' pioneered by a number of mental health workers among whom Maxwell Jones (1953, 1968) of the United Kingdom and Harry Wilmer (1958) of the USA are prominent. The therapeutic community is considered to be a setting in which the whole of the patient's time spent in hospital is thought of as treatment. The entire social resources of the hospital are mobilized in treatment and the patients are regarded as active participants and collaborators in their own therapy as well as that of the other patients and in the actual management of the hospital; this is in contrast to the traditionally passive and receptive role assigned to patients.

The social structure of the therapeutic community is felt to be markedly different from that of traditional hospital ward. The proponents of the therapeutic community consider it to be equalitarian, democratic, permissive and communal as opposed to what they consider to be the rigid, hierarchial, stereotyped and even tyrannical patterns of the traditional ward. In the therapeutic community there is a continuous detailed yet far reaching examination of the roles and role relationship of both staff and patient. For example, one item which seems to receive an enormous amount of attention in the literature of this field is the problem of the nurses' uniform. The white uniform is felt to be particularly symbolic of the old hierarchical status relationships in hospitals and the voluntary relinquishment of this badge of office by the nurse following months of discussion is invariably thought to represent an important advance in the furtherance of an equalitarian and democratic ward community.

A feature which is basic to the therapeutic community concept is the daily community meeting in which the entire staff and patient population meet together to ventilate ward problems germane to the entire group. It is felt that the upper limit for such meetings is approximately a hundred patients. The meetings are probably themselves therapeutic, but even if they are not therapy in the strict sense they represent an attempt to plan carefully patient management and to enhance other treatment methods by the mobilization of social forces in the environment.

Following the community meeting the staff meets for a so-called 'feedback' or 'post-mortem' session. It is at this meeting that the thoughts, feelings and attitudes of the staff in relationship to the preceding community meetings are examined. During these meetings many of the fears and anxieties of the staff surface and are dealt with by education and support. The staff meeting is the major vehicle for working through problems between the various staff levels such as those of physicians, nurses and ward attendants. In addition to these plenary sessions, units of this type often have a patient council involved with handling the housekeeping details of ward management. Dr Jones warns against allowing this patient council to assume too much responsibility without having staff to turn to in times of need. Otherwise the patient council will be seen by the other patients as some kind of a special and self-appointed ruling body which has taken over patient care by subterfuge.

The fundamental precept of the therapeutic community is that the patient is also a therapist who has therapeutic potentials within himself which can be encouraged and developed under constant and appropriate medical and other professional supervision. It is felt, however, that ultimate responsibilities must belong to the physicians in charge of the wards. The authority may lie fallow at times but it is always there to be exercised. Of course, in situations of changing ward composition, greater or lesser amounts of direct authority might have to be used by those in charge. For example, on a ward that has remained stable for some time with little patient inflow or outflow the community may be running at a relatively high level of effectiveness with the patients assuming a great deal of responsibility. On the other hand, the sudden transfer of a number of patients and the influx of some highly disturbed newcomers may make it necessary to re-exert more direct controls. The sharing of important responsibilities with the staff is construed as ameliorating the over dependent and unselfconfident approach which is so characteristic of hospitalized psychiatric patients. As time passes, the daily whole community meetings tend to foster increased communication between members of the community about the various emotional problems possessed by each member. Even the large size of the group does not seem to completely damp down such revelations.

The therapeutic community has many zealous supporters but it has also been subjected to strong criticism. The principal criticisms have been succinctly summarized by Dr B. B. Zeitlyn (1967). The initial criticism relates to the imprecision and ambiguities inherent in the term 'therapeutic community'. It has been used to denote treatment approaches ranging from those of traditional wards which simply have active group therapy to wards entirely run by the patients with the motivations of the staff seemingly being the major focus of concern. Other terms such as administrative therapy, social therapy or milieu therapy are sometimes used interchangeably with that of therapeutic community. Jones argues, however, that in fact it is probably healthy that there is no one model of the therapeutic community and that a multiplicity of forms should arise based upon the general principle of patient participation in the therapeutic process. Another criticism of the therapeutic community and indeed other broad social psychiatric approaches to the treatment of patients in mental hospitals is the lack of any sort of firm evidence as to the specific effectiveness of the treatment regime. That the mobilization of energy and enthusiasm of the staff attendant upon a new approach to treatment can be helpful in bringing regressed patients out of their shells is incontestable; however, one might well wish to have evidence that the treatment regime in question offers more than merely some generalized placebo affect. A research design adequate to yield evidence about the effectiveness of so comprehensive a series of changes in the environment would be extremely difficult to develop. In addition to the very real difficulties of research on such complex and heterogeneous variables there is also, unfortunately, a bias against research on the part of some 'activists'. Whatever the reasons, the fact remains that there is little hard evidence obtained in longitudinal follow-up studies to indicate clearly the specific effectiveness of any of these broad-gauged social psychiatric treatment regimes. It must also be said that it remains to be proved that all types and categories of patients are indeed made worse by standard in-patient treatment. There are now, and no doubt in the future will be, certain patients who require and enormously profit from a period of time in a regularized, structured and sheltered environment.

Finally, a central problem in the implementation of the therapeutic community and patient government approach is that of ultimate authority and ultimate responsibility. If the physician totally abdicates authority and responsibility for the direction of patient care it might well be asked of what use is he? There are problems continuously arising on any psychiatric ward which appear to require technical knowledge as well as good will for their appropriate solution. Obviously, many physicians are quite unwilling to surrender what they regard as their correct prerogatives and responsibilities in the treatment of sick patients. Even amongst those who say they are able to shed their status and rank, a suspicion remains as to whether this abrogation can really be effective. Even if the physician is not wearing a white coat there are other identifying features of his demeanour and speech which denote some separation from the rest of the group. Oddly enough, several of the most vigorous advocates of therapeutic community ventures have themselves been accused of being not so secret tyrants who, under the façade of democratic permissiveness, are able to skilfully manipulate the wards and groups to do their bidding and to expel any dissident members who do not go along with the group consensus.

It is my view that, although many of these criticisms of the therapeutic community and related concepts of milieu therapy are well taken, one must also recognize the substantial and, I think beneficial, impact such ideas have had upon the treatment of the mentally ill, particularly in regard to the prevention of the bad effects of prolonged and repressive hospitalization. This approach has certainly fostered the notion that the patient's participation in the therapeutic process might be useful for him and might help to build his confidence. The therapeutic community approach re-emphasizes the dignity of the individual patient as well as enhancing the feelings of worth on the part of often neglected staff members such as ward attendants. At its best such a regime can help to promote social interaction and better and less distorted communications between staff members and between the staff and the patients. It also introduces a generally humane note into mental hospital treatment. However, one must guard against judging such endeavours to prevent an uncritical enthusiasm for unproved methods to sweep away certain procedures which might be beneficial to the patient but which might be abhorrent to certain groups in the hospital community. For example, some nurses might object to the giving of electric shock therapy to depressed and suicidal patients. In this case a group consensus against this treatment might not be in the best interest of the individual patient. Serious, acute and life-threatening problems are usually not ones which are amenable to group decision. Napoleon was always delighted to fight against any army commanded by a council of war knowing it would invariably be timid and disorganized. Similarly, there are times in medicine and even in the psychiatric part of medicine when decisive action must be taken to help the patient. The community is ill-equipped to act *en bloc* in such events. On the other hand, these emergencies are sufficiently uncommon so that many decisions, particularly involving general ward management, can well be handled through the medium of group discussion. In any case, milieu-therapy, therapeutic communities and open wards are a feature of present-day hospital psychiatry and few would wish to turn the clock back to padded rooms, manacled patients and sadistic and aloof attendants.

8 Community Psychiatry

It seems natural enough to an epidemiologist or a public health worker to look beyond the hospital to the community from which patients come. Nevertheless, this community point of view was slow in its development in psychiatry, even though as we have already seen, dissatisfaction with therapeutic practices in mental hospitals has been manifested for a very long time. Although in America earlier in the century such phenomena as the Mental Hygiene Movement and the establishment of child guidance clinics seemed to foreshadow a growing interest in the possible prevention of mental illness, such endeavours remained extremely limited in scope. There were promising developments in such countries as Holland and the United Kingdom prior to the Second World War, for example the Mental Treatment Act of 1930 in the UK which set up psychiatric out-patient departments in general hospitals. However, there is no doubt that the war gave an enormous impetus to all sorts of movements concerned with social justice and expanded medical care. Seeds were sown at that time which later germinated into such flowers as the National Health Service in Great Britain (1948) and the establishment of the National Institute of Mental Health in the United States (1949). These institutions emphasized the right of every individual to receive high quality medical care, including psychiatric treatment if indicated. In order to bring psychiatric care to all segments of society, legislation has been passed in both the United Kingdom and the United States facilitating the establishment of community psychiatric programmes.

It might be useful at the outset to attempt to clarify just what is meant by community psychiatry, which has been described somewhat grandiosely as the third revolution in psychiatry, the other two presumably being the freeing of hospitalized mental patients from chains and the advent of psychoanalysis.

The term community psychiatry, as is the case with so many others in the field of mental health, has a certain ambiguity. Such terms as social psychiatry, preventive psychiatry, community mental health and public mental health apparently have similar meanings and are often used interchangeably. However, the term can be operationally elucidated by listing some activities which are considered to be part of community psychiatry:

1. Epidemiological studies, opinion surveys, operational analysis of community needs, resources, information, programmes and education relative to psychiatric problems.

2. The development, planning, organization, administration and operation of community programmes concerned with mental health. These programmes would include the inauguration and operation of community psychiatric hospital services, including day treatment centres, night hospitals, out-patient clinics offering emergency services, emergency clinics, psychiatric home visits, and preventive and rehabilitative services designed to prevent individuals from either entering or re-entering a mental hospital.

3. Consultations to community decision makers as well as to other agencies which provide psychiatric care. For example, in the United States, in order for a comprehensive community mental health centre to qualify for federal assistance it must offer in-patient treatment, out-patient treatment, partial hospitalization (day or night care), emergency services twenty-four hours a day, consultation and education to individual and group leaders in the community, and in its fullest development, diagnostic services, rehabilitation, after-care for hospitalized patients, training for professional mental health workers and others, as well as research and evaluation.

We will now examine these various aspects of community psychiatry in greater detail. That part of community psychiatry which is most clearly allied to general clinical psychiatry is the provision of community-based mental health facilities which treat people in a setting closer to their homes than would be the case in a large and possibly remote mental hospital. Examples of such facilities would be day hospitals, night hospitals or walk-in clinics all of which are facilities which ensure that the patient does not face the choice between complete hospitalization or no treatment at all. These institutions provide care for patients who do not seem to require the total isolation from the community given by the traditional mental hospital. For example, in the day hospital the patient might receive group psychotherapy, occupational therapy, recreational therapy, or even somatic treatment such as electro-shock therapy during the day but will return home at night, allowing him daily access to the community and a continuing contact with his family which would be lost if he were hospitalized at some distance from his home.

Similarly, the night hospital allows the patient to work and be in the community during the day and to receive hospitalization at night. The advantages claimed for these types of partial hospitalization include economic savings, the maintenance of the patient's ties to his family and community, and the less serious image of his illness imparted by his remaining to some degree in the community rather than being completely isolated in some mysterious asylum. The walk-in clinic (also known as the crisis clinic or emergency clinic or similar names) is another community psychiatric service. In America the rationale for such a clinic is usually said to rest upon the work of Gerald Caplan (1964) of the Harvard School of Public Health, particularly on his emphasis of the frequency and importance of temporary crises in a patient's life which can be dealt with most successfully by early and brief psychiatric treatment. Caplan delineates a preventive orientation aimed towards the reduction of the amount of disability and defect in a given population. He speaks of primary, secondary and tertiary prevention. By primary prevention is meant a reduction in the incidence of a disease by preventing its occurrence. Thus we prevent water-borne enteric infections by chlorination of the water. Correspondingly, if certain environmental features could be proved to cause psychiatric disease, their removal might result in primary prevention of psychiatric disability. Secondary prevention involves the early identification of the sick so they might be treated rapidly to prevent further disability. This corresponds to vigorous case finding and prompt treatment. An example might be mass screening for tuberculosis with the immediate treatment of individuals identified by the demonstration of lesions on x-ray films. Similarly, in psychiatry secondary prevention might be established by providing readily available services to treat rapidly individuals at the beginning of an episode of severe mental or emotional disturbance in order to prevent progression of the disorder into a full-blown psychosis. Tertiary prevention is the rehabilitation of the already disabled so as to reduce the degree of disability. In general medicine this would correspond, for example, to rehabilitative services for those crippled with poliomyelitis. In psychiatry, tertiary prevention might involve post-hospital care for chronic schizophrenic patients in an attempt to allow them to live useful lives within the community.

The emergency clinic attempts to deal with short-term, acute problems in the life of an individual which temporarily overwhelm his coping capacities. As has been previously mentioned, the armed forces have long provided such emergency psychiatric services as close to the individual's unit as possible in both peace and war.

Similar clinics of an emergency type in the United Kingdom have come into being in quite a pragmatic way to answer the need for swift and focused treatment of the innumerable people who are in the midst of severe emotional upheavals in their lives and who need some form of prompt help. The major features of such clinics are their lack of a waiting list so that the patient receives treatment immediately; the brevity of the psychotherapy, encompassing at most a few visits; its concentration on present problems rather than on the childhood antecedents, if any, of the patient's present difficulties; a flexibility of technique; and an optimism of outlook.

Obviously the combination of day hospital, night hospital, emergency clinic, rehabilitation centre, out-patient department, follow-up clinic, acute treatment centre for alcoholism and drug addiction, and so forth, into one united facility known as a comprehensive mental health centre or a community mental health centre appears to offer substantial advantages (and perhaps some dangers as well). Centres of this genre have been in existence for some time in the United Kingdom. An example of such a centre known to the author is the one at Horsham, Sussex, called the St Christopher's Day Hospital. It is an integral part of a mental health care system including also the Graylingwell Hospital serving patients from Horsham, Crawley and surrounding districts. It operates twenty-four hours a day with a constant staff of four including one full-time psychiatrist of registrar status and one part-time psychiatric registrar. In addition a psychiatrist of consultant status is available at all times. The centre has an occupational therapist, nurses of both sexes and a social worker as well. Patients may come for out-patient visits, electric shock treatment, drug treatments, group therapy, occupational therapy and day hospital care.

When the centre was inaugurated, all the general practitioners within the general area served by it were told of its existence, its mode of operation and that they must refer their psychiatric patients to the centre, rather than directly to the Graylingwell Hospital. After the patients are referred to the unit there are several possible paths of action available to the staff. First, if the case seems urgent, they make an immediate home visit. Second, if some urgency exists, but to a lesser degree than that requiring a home visit, the patient is seen at the centre that day. If the problem does not seem at all urgent an appointment is made for an out-patient visit at a later date. This comprehensive yet selective approach ensures that everyone will be seen and carefully evaluated prior to any possible admission to the mental hospital. After a patient is evaluated there are various dispositional possibilities. First, it may be recommended that the patient receive treatment at home; second, treatment at the day centre; third, out-patient treatment by means of a regular or an irregular appointment schedule; fourth, he may be recommended for admission to Graylingwell Hospital; or fifth, no treatment may be deemed necessary. The staff at such a centre is extraordinarily dedicated, enthusiastic and very knowledgeable about the minutest details of local conditions. This is in contrast to some units in the United States where most of the staff are professionals coming from elsewhere who do not possess a really profound understanding of local conditions. Moreover, a city like Los Angeles has an extraordinarily mobile population which may turn over a number of times within a decade so that perhaps no one can be said to know a given district of Los Angeles in the same detailed and profound way that one might be said to know a portion of Shropshire or West Sussex.

The Horsham Centre has been intimately involved with research since its inception. In view of the long history in psychiatry, and indeed in medicine in general, of enthusiastically received new treatment forms gradually falling into disuse because of their ineffectiveness, it is clearly essential that research and operational analyses be incorporated in the design of new therapeutic plans. Unfortunately this dictum has by no means received full acceptance in America. However, the work at the Horsham Centre has been under the constant scrutiny of the Medical Research Council's Clinical Psychiatry Research Unit, Graylingwell Hospital, Chichester, Sussex, ably directed by Dr Peter Sainsbury.

The work carried on in Sussex by Grad and Sainsbury (1966, 1969) was designed to evaluate the effects of the so-called 'Worthing Experiment' and its sequelae. This experiment was begun by Dr J. Carse, formerly Superintendent of the Graylingwell Hospital, in the late 1950s and was occasioned by the progressive rise in admissions to the hospital to such a level that gross overcrowding had occurred. Carse and others evolved a scheme whereby a very active out-patient service would be available in the town of Worthing. The inhabitants of this town were heavy contributors to the patient load at Graylingwell. This out-patient service would try as vigorously as possible to prevent the admission of patients to the hospital and attempt to treat them in their home setting.

The experiment was a marked success if measured by the sole criterion of diminished hospital admissions from the

Worthing area. This scheme of local mental health centres was then greatly expanded and centres were placed in other areas of West Sussex.

In this evaluation of the Worthing Experiment and of the other subsequently developed mental health centres, four main questions were asked:

1. Who is referred to the psychiatric service in an area which has introduced community care? In other words, what are the referral rates for patients in different social and clinical groups?

2. Who is admitted to the hospital when there is a community service, and similarly, what social and clinical factors determine whether the patient is treated at home, in a hospital or elsewhere? Community care presupposes that factors other than clinical ones, for example, community attitudes and social and family situations, impinge upon the decision as to whether or not patients are admitted to hospital. Grad and Sainsbury were especially interested in examining conditions favouring particular types of patient disposition.

3. What are the effects on the family of caring for a mentally ill member at home? A universal criticism of community care programmes is that they might impose an unfair burden on the family, a burden better assumed by the mental hospital.

4. How does the outcome of the patient's illness in a community service compare with the outcome when treatment is given in hospital?

Obviously in addition to these four formal questions, there are other areas of interest which might emerge from the data, for example, information about the kind of services which might be required by families with members undergoing community care.

A research design was constructed in which representative samples of patient populations referred to either a community service or to a hospital based service were compared. The plan required a means of collecting reliable and valid data on the factors believed to be related to the problems they were attempting to study. Pertinent data included accurate and objective assessments of the patients' clinical state, their social characteristics, and their family circumstances.

The Old Manor Hospital in Salisbury, Wiltshire, was chosen to provide the comparison group not only because of the propinquity of Salisbury but also because it is a town not too dissimilar in size to Chichester (35,000 v. 20,000) and even more similar in spirit, down to the common details of a market cross and a handsome cathedral. In fact, it was shown that the Salisbury (and other Wiltshire) patients were demographically and clinically closely similar to the Chichester (and other Sussex towns) group save only that there were more old people in the Chichester sample than in the Salisbury one because of the large number of older individuals living directly on the South Coast in retirement enclaves. The staff–patient ratio was similar in both Salisbury and Chichester. There were more social work services available in Salisbury. The principal difference between the two areas in terms of psychiatric facilities was, indeed, the one variable crucial to the study, namely, that in Salisbury there was no community mental health centre. Hence, patients were referred directly to the hospital by their local physicians, whereas in Chichester the new experimental mental health centres were established.

Research proceded as follows: first, for one year codified information on all patients referred in the West Sussex area and seen by Graylingwell Hospital personnel was obtained. This was accomplished by the means of structured interviews using extremely elaborate interview schedules which delineated the patients' demographic features and clinical status *in extenso*. Identical information was obtained on the control or comparison group of patients who were the responsibility of the Old Manor Hospital in Salisbury.

Then in both populations one in three random samples were chosen, and in addition to data gathered on the patient himself, a principal investigator, Dr Jacqueline Grad, went to the homes of the patients and talked to family informants as well as to the local physician. A scale was constructed which very elaborately measured the effects of the patient's mental illness on the family's income, on the children in the home, on the family's social activities, on household routine, and on nursing care. A two-year follow-up was obtained in which the patient and family status were rated by the patient, by the family, by the attending psychiatrist, the research psychiatrist and the general practitioner. There was an attempt made to match a Chichester case (what is known in epidemiology as the proband) with a control case in Salisbury matched on such variables as severity of illness, burden to the family, and frequency of certain symptoms.

The results of the study showed that the annual referral rate to Chichester services (6·8/1000) was higher than in the Salisbury area (5·3/1000). This higher rate in Chichester was maintained for all ages, sex, marital status, social and diagnostic categories; more patients of every kind were therefore referred to the community service as compared to the pure hospital service. This was particularly true for the aged, the lower classes, the depressed, those living alone and those with organic psychoses. The patients seen in Chichester tended to have been ill a shorter time before being seen than was the case in Salisbury. These data do seem to indicate that if one provides a community health centre, one can expect a greater rate of referral to psychiatric services than in locales where a mental hospital programme alone exists. This referral rate must not be confused with admission to the hospital rate which, as might be expected, was far higher in Salisbury than in Chichester. For example, 52 per cent of all patients referred to psychiatric services by general practitioners in Salisbury were initially admitted to the mental hospital, whereas only 18 per cent of those in Chichester were initially admitted. In Chichester, the remaining 82 per cent were taken care of by the community centres or received no treatment. Over a two-year period 62 per cent of the Chichester patients remained in the community exclusively, compared to 41 per cent in Salisbury.

In the admission of patients to the hospital both in Salisbury and Chichester, social considerations were often more important than purely clinical ones. To be sure, symptoms such as overt aggressiveness and suicidal threats would make admission to hospital more likely; however, income level and home situation as well as age also played a large role in the decision for admission to hospital. The composition of the family and the level of problems (other than the patient's illness) in the home was assessed prior to the decision for admission. In some patient categories, for example among neurotics, the disturbance to the family by the patient remaining in the home rather than being hospitalized seemed to be greater in the Chichester than in the Salisbury group. However, this increased family burden might well be related to inadequate social service support for certain patients. Certainly it is clear that a really well organized, adequately staffed and efficient community service can maintain a majority of psychiatric patients in the community without adverse affect on their clinical course. It is not quite so clear at present that there may not be an adverse affect on other family members, such as children, of having a mentally ill patient treated at home rather than in the mental hospital. It is extraordinarily difficult to measure the possible long-term and perhaps subtle deleterious effects of a psychiatrically ill person on the rest of his family, but they might be considerable. This question remains to be finally resolved.

The establishment of comprehensive mental health centres located within communities and treating patients away from large residential mental hospitals has aroused relatively little controversy, but not so the staffing and control of such centres. For example, some social workers, particularly in the USA, resent what they regard as psychiatric intrusion into the areas of community organization and community problems which they have long regarded as their own occupational provinces. Similarly, some clinical and social psychologists have objected strenuously to the idea that the mental health centre must always be headed by a psychiatrist. In turn, certain psychiatrists have objected to the placing of non-psychiatrists, such as psychologists and social workers, in policy-making positions within the mental health centre. Finally, some of the centres in the United States, particularly in slum areas, have been split by extreme dissension resulting from conflicts between the views of the professional staff and the views of various boards of laymen from the surrounding community who have been engaged to help formulate the policies and operational procedures of the clinics. Some of these battles have even made headlines in medical newspapers and have resulted in the expulsion of certain staff.

The controversies about community mental health centres are, however, as nothing compared to the polemical struggles about the use of mental health consultants, particularly psychiatrists, to advise and guide various community organizations in an attempt to bring about the primary prevention of psychiatric disorders. The roles of the mental health consultant are envisioned as ranging from ones which are clearly in the medical tradition such as consultations with school nurses or public health departments, to the essentially non-medical role of advisor to political decision makers about matters of public policy such as housing or recreational facilities.

Zuithoff (1969), advisor to the Ministry of Cultural Affairs and Social Welfare and the Ministry of Justice in The Hague, has cogently described the principal tasks and problems of the psychiatric consultant to administrative organizations. He has consulted with the Ministry of Social Welfare about such important social problems as generational conflicts, the problems of the youth, the family, minority groups, the poor and the influence of rapid social changes on the basic units of society. To the Ministry of Justice he has offered consultation in such areas as the understanding of delinquency, social deviance and the training of individuals to work in correctional and rehabilitative settings for juvenile delinquents and adult criminals. Essentially he offers a viewpoint from the behavioural sciences, particularly community psychiatry, to be incorporated into the decision-making process of the Ministry. This job of advisor is a very difficult one and the individual and his advice tend to be met with great resistance. Resistance appears to be best overcome by a combination of tact, inter-personal skills and, perhaps most importantly, the demonstration that one's advice is sound and is based on a foundation of solid and substantial knowledge. Epidemiological follow-up and pilot studies which develop specific data bearing on the actual effect of a given social change can be very helpful in the maintenance of a continuing programme which will survive successfully after the first surge of enthusiasm for an innovation dies down. Political organizations being what they are, an advisor whose advice doesn't seem to work out or one whose advice seems to be based mainly on his own theories or ideological biases without being buttressed by solid evidence generally exerts little lasting influence.

How one views the activity of a psychiatrist acting as an advisor to organizations remaking society depends perhaps on one's ideological viewpoint. Professor Melvin Sabshin (1969) believes that there are major ideological groupings among psychiatrists which he and his colleagues characterize as the 'psychotherapeutic, the somatotherapeutic and sociotherapeutic ideologies'. The psychotherapeutic and somatotherapeutic purist are both opposed to the growing 'community mental health movement'. The somatotherapeutic purist, in Professor Sabshin's view, tends to think purely in medical models. He is disturbed by the vague definitions of social psychiatrists; the use by social psychiatrists of models other than the medical one; and the seemingly mindless activism of some community mental health advocates. The psychotherapeutic purist sees community mental health centres as dispensing dilute and superficial treatment to a great mass of people without really giving thorough treatment to any one person. Similarly, he regards the social theories of the causation of mental illness as naïve and lamentably lacking in substantiating evidence. In the purist view, the community psychiatrist seems to pay little attention to the clinical knowledge of such entities as the unconscious, painstakingly developed over the last seventy years.

Unfortunately the merits of many programmes are already being obscured in various *ad hominem* arguments of great vituperation. Although traducing one's enemy is by no means unknown in other spheres of activity, psychiatric quarrels typically revert to the questioning of the motivation of one's opponents and labelling their objections as 'resistance', 'neurotic', or in the case of the social psychiatric programmes, 'reactionary', 'socialistic', and so forth. Unfortunately, in the ensuing tumult the substantative issues are often obscured.

There are certainly powerful arguments to be put forward justifying psychiatric services at a local level, perhaps connected administratively with the hospital system and offering a panoply of therapeutic and rehabilitative measures. Some o these activities which conform neither to the traditional psychotherapeutic or to the traditional medical model might still be of benefit to large numbers of suffering people. To serve the suffering, is, after all the highest charge to the medical profession and the realization of this ideal must not be hampered by adherence to past definitions of proper medical concerns, if such definitions are really no longer useful.

The case for psychiatrists involving themselves in social planning is movingly and forcibly stated by Matthew Dumont (1968) in his book *The Absurd Healer: Perspectives of a Community Psychiatrist*. Dumont involved himself closely with political figures, social workers, community leaders of all types, city planners, architects and other interested citizens in an attempt to alter the social and physical conditions of certain urban slums. Dumont worked with people who dwelt in these areas, both young and old, as well as with those who were involved with the control or change of conditions in the total environment. Dumont described how public health measures must be shaped to fit local conditions, for example, he induced the bartender of a local tavern catering for elderly men, all of whom were lonely, alcoholic and low on vitamins, to dispense vitamin pills with the beer. He is only one of many who have described the difficulties of developing useful and permanent programmes in slum areas. Even services which initially begin as purely medical ventures are quickly involved in social problems such as housing, unemployment, inadequate schools and policy–community relationships. Scherl and English (1969) indicate that in addition to therapeutic services for the mentally ill which must be hand tailored to suit local conditions, comprehensive health centres in urban slums must also offer educational programmes on such topics as health and nutrition. The centre must also involve the residents of the community themselves in the planning and delivery of health services or it will fail to carry out its mission.

These publications are but a few examples amongst many which plead most strongly the case for psychiatrists to involve themselves directly in the reorganization of society. It appears to many who work in the slums that a rather complete social reorganization must take place if the manifold injustices they witness are to be irradicated. Some psychiatrists advocate moving beyond mere consultative help with city governments, the school system, the police and the judiciary, to active attempts, in the name of community psychiatry, to alter society in a substantive way. In the United States and to a lesser degree in the United Kingdom such activities of community psychiatry in slum areas are complicated by the question of race and there are currently considerable arguments about whether race should be considered in the appointment of the mental health professionals to posts in centres serving primarily black communities. I think at present it is the consensus of black psychiatrists in the USA that race should indeed be a primary consideration in such appointments and that in the future both institutions serving the black community, and investigations in that community should be staffed primarily by blacks. The writings of Pierce (1969) and Pinderhughes (1969) emphasize the need for this policy if social psychiatry is to play its envisaged role in the sort of radical social change they believe essential in slum areas.

On the other hand, there is quite reasonable and substantial concern about the obscurity of the goals and the paucity of theories and concepts in the community mental health field. There is also the very real problem of the appropriate use of trained manpower. There is no doubt that a few psychiatrists view themselves, at least in fantasy, as a potential Richelieu sitting at the elbow of powerful men and remaking society. Apart from this small group of people with grandiose views, there are a large number of psychiatrists humbly and devotedly engaged in all kinds of direct community and social action. Many professionals have already raised questions as to whether, in fact, psychiatric training confers any special expertise in effecting beneficial social change or, perhaps more to the point, if there are to be individuals functioning in this capacity, whether the traditional training of the psychiatrist really is the best possible education for this role. After all, a psychiatrist is trained first as a general physician and his subsequent psychiatric training at present takes primarily a medical approach. Whether or not ten to twelve years of training in the medical area following graduation from secondary school is the best preparation for a political or quasi-political role is something which might well be seriously challenged. It might be far better to develop a specific training programme for those who were going to fulfill this kind of role, one in which they might receive more exposure to history, economics, political science, sociology, philosophy, and rather less to anatomy, molecular biology, etc., than is the case in the present medical curriculum. If there are to be meaningful and important contributions to public policy by psychiatric consultants then they must be able to offer the fruits of appropriate education and experience. Dr Bertram S. Brown (1969) himself the Director, National Institute of Mental Health, and an extremely important figure in the development of the community mental health centre programme has indicated that psychiatric input is needed in the formulation of public policy in areas such as penology, family planning or the care of the aged, all of which require medical involvement. This consultative function is surely important enough to necessitate psychiatrists of enormous knowledge, wisdom and competence being available to perform in this way. However, there is a limited supply of psychiatrists everywhere and the proper utilization of such highly trained and expensive manpower is an important question. I would venture to say that most psychiatrists will, for the forseeable future, still prefer to operate within the general medical framework and spend their time in directly treating patients. There will be, however, a minority who have the interest and the necessary resilience of personality and skills to be involved not only in the reorganization of psychiatric and health services but also in wider social planning.

At present community psychiatry is in a fluid and even a fermenting state. One must thus expect turmoil, conflict, raised voices and a clash of ideas. The precise outlines of future syntheses are blurred. One may hope that what emerges will somehow bring better health care to all members of society.

9 Conclusion

By this point, the persevering reader will doubtless have discovered that the field of social psychiatry is laden with both complexities and contradictions. This book can perhaps best serve as a prolegomenon to the study of the influence of social and other environmental factors on mental disease. The various studies cited are intended to be illustrative rather than inclusive. There are many many other studies of equal merit which might have been referred to with equal pertinence; however, this volume would have then approached encyclopedic size. One may hope that the major issues and research approaches in social psychiatry have been delineated. A detailed examination of the methods by which certain studies were conducted should acquaint the reader with the difficulties and compromises necessary in any study of humans under naturalistic conditions and should make him better able to gauge how much credence he should put in the final results of such work. Finally, it is to be hoped that those with a serious and extended interest in this field will return to the many original works cited in the bibliography for an opportunity to view in depth and detail the important contributions of the various investigators.

It might now be useful to summarize briefly the major themes developed in the preceding chapters before ending with some speculations about future trends.

We began by describing the phenomenon of unequal disease distribution. Diseases show differential prevalences in people of varying ages, races, sex, occupation and locale. Even amongst people of the same age, race, sex and occupation, all living in the same place, there are marked differences in the incidence of various diseases. That branch of science which deals with the differential distributions of diseases is known as epidemiology. Epidemiology is of great usefulness in medicine, public health and also in the field of psychiatry. It is a science based on other disciplines such as demography, statistics, clinical medicine and pathology. Demography defines the characteristics of the populations at risk for a given disease; statistics specifies the procedures by which enumeration and analyses precede; and clinical medicine and pathology provide the necessary definition of what is to be counted as a case of a given disease.

The work of Dr John Snow in the 1850s in London on epidemic cholera was examined in detail as a clear illustration of the power of the epidemiological method to help clarify the mode of transmission of a given disease and to set the stage for its possible prevention. Although he worked at a time when the bacteriological cause of cholera was as yet undiscovered, his demonstration of the pathogenic quality of faecally contaminated water led to the obvious preventive measure of decontamination of the water supply. All epidemiological investigations which seek to demonstrate differing disease rates in various populations must of necessity have some clear definition (in so far as this is possible) of what constitutes a case. Throughout history diseases have been conceptualized in various ways but certainly in recent centuries they have been viewed as entities which disrupt normal body functioning.

There has always been some difficulty in placing mental disease in the ordinary categories of medical illnesses. Some authorities have even denied that mental illnesses exist and others have thought that these aberrations in thinking, emotionality or behaviour were merely variations of normal functioning. Nevertheless, all sciences require a taxonomy and various classifications of psychiatric illness based primarily on behavioural characteristics of patients have been constructed, although other data such as the patient's history may also be taken into account. A common classification of mental illness includes such entities as psychoses which represent severe mental illnesses in which there is an impairment of the patient's reality testing and other mental functioning; neuroses which involve milder impairments of an emotional nature; and personality disorders which represent perennial behaviour patterns which seem to be maladaptive. Using classificatory schemes primarily of the descriptive type, various investigators have attempted to construct an epidemiology of mental illness. They initially relied on statistics of hospitalization to give them a notion as to the commonness of mental disease in a given locale or in a given subpopulation. Hospitalization rates, however, have been shown to reflect many factors other than disease prevalence. For example, the availability of hospital beds, legal codes relative to insanity and to commitment in mental hospitals, the cost of hospitalization, the availability of alternative health resources, the community's attitude towards mental hospitalization, and a wide variety of other social factors all affect the rate of hospitalization. In the past, because of the chronic nature of most mental illnesses and because of therapeutic attitudes regarding discharge on the part of the staff, patients tended to accumulate in mental hospitals; however, in recent years early discharge has been the rule, particularly since the widespread usage of psychotropic drugs began. Psychosis admission rates to hospital have been shown to be remarkably constant over a long period of time. In fact, there is evidence to suggest that where schizophrenia is concerned there has been no real change in the incidence rate for as long a time as adequate statistics have been available. Admission rates, of course, differ for the young as opposed to the old, male $v.$ female and for the married as opposed to the divorced or the single. In an attempt to supplement hospital statistics, various surveys have been carried out in an effort to gauge the prevalence of mental illness in the community amongst individuals who have not entered hospital for treatment. Field surveys have been carried out in a number of locales, including two major studies in Manhattan, New York, and in a rural country of Nova Scotia. These surveys attempted to interview a random selection of individuals within a given population in order to ascertain how many showed symptoms of mental illness which psychiatric judges would rate as indicating the presence of impairment due to mental disease. These data complemented the figures of treated patients arrived at by examining hospital and physician office statistics. In both instances, a significant proportion of the population, amounting to almost a quarter of the total, was felt to be significantly incapacitated or impaired by psychiatric symptoms. In Nova Scotia, communities which showed evidence of sociocultural disintegration appeared to have a greater percentage of individuals with psychiatric impairment than did communities with considerable stability and cohesiveness.

An extremely important variable in differential disease prevalence is that of social class. Social class is a heterogeneous variable encompassing vast differences in life styles between the various social classes. Social class differentials have also been demonstrated in mental illness. The work of Hollingshead and Redlich in New Haven, Connecticut, is a case in point. They performed a painstaking study in an attempt to establish a point prevalence of treated mental illness within the city, based primarily on hospitalization and physicians' records. They also conducted a sociological and demographic survey of the area and placed a sample of individuals within a five-class social structure ranging from class 1, an upper-class group of the well-to-do and high professional categories, to class 5, a group of primarily semi-skilled or unskilled labourers. They were able to demonstrate clearly an excess of treated mental diseases of the psychotic variety in social class 5.

The nature of the treatment given any psychiatric patient seemed also to differ according to his position in the class structure. Prolonged psychotherapy was given almost exclusively to upper-class patients whereas organic methods of therapy, such as electro-shock, were more frequently used in the lower-class patients. The class 5 patients who were psychotic were disproportionately represented in the sub-group who became chronic state hospital patients. Follow-up studies ten years later again showed that lower-class patients, in contrast to upper-class ones, tended to spend far more time in hospital even if the lower-class patient in question showed less evidence of psychological impairment than did his upper-class counterpart.

Many studies have shown that individuals living in depressed or 'skid-row' areas in the central portion of a large metropolis have higher rates of psychosis than do individuals of similar demographic characteristics living in areas located further towards the periphery of the city. There has been much controversy about the question as to whether such mentally ill individuals living in the central city sprang from families of similar low social status, or whether such individuals had originally come from a higher social class, and because of a mental disease which precluded their functioning effectively in society had drifted downward to end up living in a depressed area. There is evidence on both sides of this question. A number of explanations have been offered to account for the higher prevalence of mental disease in the lowest class. Some have favoured the notion that stresses of life amongst the poor have given rise to psychotic illnesses without, however, specifying precisely what the stresses were which gave rise to psychosis. In general terms the stresses spoken about are ones such as insanitary housing, gross overcrowding, no money in the family, blighted family life, omnipresent crime, alcoholism and bad education. Disturbed interactions between the members of the family from which the patient came have been pointed out as favouring the development of later psychosis. Other authorities have advanced the notion of a genetic predisposition to psychosis amongst the lower class resulting from a form of social selection in which either the patient with an inherited tendency towards mental illness, or some progenitor of his, has drifted downwards because of the hardships of mental illness to the bottom rung of the social ladder. Naturally those of the unitary bent of mind would think that there might be some validity in all these explanations. For example, there might be an accumulation of genetically predisposed individuals in the most depressed groups in society on whom the stresses of unemployment, bad nutrition, rampant crime and malevolent family relationships all operate in an additive way to increase the actual appearance of diagnosable mental disease.

In addition to the long-range effects of such factors as genetic predisposition to mental illness, disturbed family relationships during childhood or gross environmental stress incident to poverty, there are clearly some short-term phenomena which may be proximately involved in the development of emotional illness. For example, prior to the development of certain types of mental depressions, the patient will invariably be found to have suffered a severe loss, either of a person close to him or in some other important area of his life such as occupation or self-esteem. It has been shown that a high level of life changes occurring in close temporal relationship to each other predispose an individual to the development of illnesses, including mental ones. At a time when an individual feels insecure, ungratified, incompetent, helpless, hopeless or unhappy, he is maximally vulnerable to the onset of disease.

Large-scale catastrophes such as war or severe economic depression may also increase the incidence of mental illness but only in certain categories. Some types of mental illness show no change at all in incidence rate or may even decline during war while others, particularly of the psychoneurotic, psychosomatic or depressive variety may show marked increases. Overwhelming environmental stress such as seen in prolonged combat or during incarceration in a concentration camp may result in not only short-term but also chronic disturbances characterized by anxiety, insomnia, depression and many psychosomatic manifestations. Suicide rates also reflect changing social conditions and differ from one nation to another as well as between different sexes, races and age groups.

The question often arises as to whether cultures other than those of the West, in particular traditional or primitive ones, are free from mental illness. It would certainly appear from the careful studies that have been done in various cultures that mental illness is indeed ubiquitous although differing, of course, in relative frequency in various areas of the world.

For example, Lin in his sound study of mental illness in Formosa (1953), was able to show that the order of magnitude of mental illness was similar to that in the West and that the major types of mental illness recognizable in Europe or North America were recognizable in the Chinese society as well.

Similarly studies in the isolated communities of an agricultural type such as the Hutterites of the US and Canada, show that even such earth-bound communities have a significant amount of mental illness. Although mental illness is universal, the type and form of its symptoms differ markedly between cultures. Schizophrenic patients from various national groups differ in the amount of activity and the types and quality of delusions, hallucinations and bizarre behaviour shown. This is particularly striking in areas like Hawaii, where the State Mental Hospital has patients of many different ethnic origins. However, there appears to be a core of psychiatric manifestations that is common to all the groups.

In addition to differences in the patients themselves there are also differences in diagnostic styles between the psychiatrists of various nations and even between the psychiatrists of the same nation. However, in most studies the amount of diagnostic agreement between psychiatrists as to the major category into which a patient should be fitted is greater than chance, often impressively so.

In the past there were described a number of stereotyped psychiatric syndromes found amongst non-industrialized people such as Malays, Eskimos and American Indians. These appeared to be syndromes in which the manifestations were directly shaped by cultural pressures and cultural sanctions. As the societies which harboured these phenomena have changed under the impact of Westernization, these peculiar illnesses have tended to disappear. Cultures obviously shape the expression of mental illness through their child-rearing practices, indoctrinations, sanctions, encouragements and discouragements.

Along with an interest in the amount and type of mental illness within the community, there has been also a concentration of social psychiatric research on the problems of hospital psychiatry. Investigators and reformers have agreed that conditions in the past in many of the large mental hospitals were so deplorable that these institutions actually exerted a deleterious effect on the course of the patient's mental illness rather than being therapeutic. Various types of hospital were described in the course of which the institution was seen to have played an important role by fostering passivity, dependency and retrogressive behaviour. In addition to the adverse psychological effects of an overcrowded, understaffed and custodial environment, a high incidence of infectious diseases and malnutrition was also noted. Other descriptive works have focused upon social interactions in mental hospitals, particularly those amongst the staff involving vital decisions on patient care. It has been shown that staff conflict and staff disagreement, particularly of the covert type, may result in exacerbations of the condition of many patients within the institution. Critics of an extreme type have even placed mental hospitals into a category of 'total institutions' in company with prisons, military barracks and concentration camps; in this view patients are regarded as inmates who are robbed of their individuality and who must conform to a certain set of doctrines or never be released. However, particularly in the years since the end of the Second World War, there have been many liberating movements in mental hospital management. Various terms have been applied to these efforts, the most popular of which is 'therapeutic community'. The fundamental idea of the therapeutic community is that the patient has potentialities to help not only in his own recovery but also in the treatment of other patients. The community attempts to lower the barriers between patients and staff and to increase communication flow. Although many criticisms have been levelled at the notion of the therapeutic community, particularly in regard to the vagueness of its concepts and definitions and to the possibility it offers to diffusion of authority and chaotic patient management; nevertheless, the spirit which underlies this enterprise has brought a much more humane atmosphere to many hospitals than existed there in the past.

Not only have there been internal reforms within the mental hospital, but also there have been many changes in the methods of delivering psychiatric care to the community. A new sub-speciality of psychiatry called community psychiatry has arisen. Community psychiatry deals particularly with the development, organization and operation of community psychiatric services and also with consultations to decision makers in the community about programmes to do with matters such as housing or assistance to the aged, which impinge upon the mental health of its members. Community psychiatry also embraces the epidemiological and operational analysis of community needs, resources and programmes.

Centres of a comprehensive type have been built in various areas to provide: partial hospitalization for psychiatric patients, in-patient treatment, out-patient treatment, twenty-four-hour-a-day emergency services, consultative services and rehabilitative services. The precise shape and functioning of any given clinic is influenced not only by the policies of the medical founders but also by the rules of the government agency which supplies funds and by various social forces within the community itself. Obviously, there have been and will continue to be numerous conflicts about the organization and management of such centres. At their best they can be shown to prevent hospitalization for many people who are in need of psychiatric help but for whom hospitalization would be deleterious. Prior to the establishment of such centres individuals in this category had either to consult a private psychiatrist or if they lacked sufficient funds to do so they either had to enter hospital or be without treatment at all. Careful follow-up studies of community mental health centres in the United Kingdom have shown that they are highly successful in preventing hospitalization and in rendering valuable help to many individuals within the community.

An area of greater controversy is that of mental health consultation. In its most medical form, for example, consultation to public health nurses, or to a school system on mental hygiene, it is regarded by virtually all as unexceptionable. In its more activist form it is less highly regarded by many segments of medicine. There are those, who from their experiences in community psychiatry, feel that if there is to be prevention of certain kinds of mental, behavioural or emotional disturbances there must be some radical reorganizations of society. These individuals feel that community psychiatrists should have a valuable role as advisors to politicians and other decision makers in the shaping of a new type of society which would be more conducive to good mental health throughout the population than is the case with any present society. This activist few is regarded with scepticism by large and influential segments of psychiatry.

Few men can discern the outlines of the future, even in their own field. This is particularly true if one tries to move beyond the mere extrapolation of present trends to the foreseeing of unexpected developments. The author claims no prophetic powers but is willing to think about some future directions of psychiatry. At the time of writing this volume it is clear there are two areas in which there is enormous interest and great change. The first is the whole field of social psychiatry which we have touched upon in this book; the other is the biological basis of psychiatry, including chemical studies of brain processes as well as psychopharmacology. Enormous strides are being made in the biochemical aspects of psychiatry, but enough is already known for all to realize that we are merely on the first leg of a very, very long journey indeed, and that many decades of sailing lie ahead before the destination of precise knowledge of the chemical mediation of psychiatric diseases is reached. When that day comes and come it must, not only will we have a clearer picture of the mode of transmission of mental diseases but also, it is to be hoped, we shall have much more precise and specific methods of prevention and treatment.

On the other flank of the attack, so to speak, is the whole area of social and community influences on mental aberrations. In the practical sphere, the community health movement will doubtless come to a full blossoming and then suffer the fate of all movements. That is, it will become regularized, no doubt will contract somewhat and probably lose much of its present excitement. One would hope that research in this area would now move from the general to the specific.

There perhaps will also be continuing changes in public attitudes towards mental disease. Certainly the attitudes of the past (and the present) have been those of ignorance, fear, apprehension and rejection. In recent years there has been some change or shift in public attitudes towards greater understanding and acceptance. Nevertheless, within certain segments of society the old feelings still prevail. In the future it is to be hoped that what might be considered a rational and humane attitude, based on accurate knowledge of a simple kind about mental disorders, will prevail throughout society. However, the emotional and attitudinal barriers to this development are very great and should never be underestimated.

Other developments will include a much better specification of the optimum pattern of treatment for the particular patient so that truly individualized care will be available. The evidence on which such therapeutic approaches will be based will have been obtained by a variety of clinical, basic science and epidemiological studies. There may well be in the future many different categories of non-medical personnel who will render various forms of psychiatric care, including psychotherapy. Computer and laboratory methods assisting in diagnosis and patient management will be extensively available.

As time passes there will be many social changes – some planned, some not – which, in affecting the incidence of certain kinds of mental disorders, will give us clues to the intricate and subtle interaction between social forces and mental disease.

We end this 'strange eventful history' with a challenge. There are many Lake Victorias of social psychiatry awaiting discovery. Our explorations have barely left the coast. There is still much to be discovered and much work to be done. Let those who see social psychiatry as confused and obscure, take up the endeavour to bring order and clarity to one map of this rich territory.

References

ABRAHAM, K. (1912), 'Notes on the psychoanalytical investigation and treatment of manic-depressive insanity and allied conditions', in *Selected Papers on Psychoanalysis*, Basic Books and Hogarth Press, 1953.

ADAMS, H. B. (1964), 'Mental illness or interpersonal behavior?' *Amer. Psychol.*, vol. 19, no. 3, pp. 191–7.

AMERICAN PSYCHIATRIC ASSOCIATION (1968), *Diagnostic and Statistical Manual of Mental Disorders*, 2nd edn.

ARTHUR, R. J. (1965), 'Stability in psychosis admission rates: three decades of Navy experience', *Public Health Reports*, vol. 80, no. 6, pp. 512–14.

BETTELHEIM, B. (1960), *The Informed Heart*, Free Press.

BOCKOVEN, J. S. (1963), *Moral Treatment in American Psychiatry*, Springer Publishing Co.

BRIDGMAN, P. W. (1927), *The Logic of Modern Physics*, Macmillan Co.

BROWN, B. S. (1968), 'Psychiatric practice and public policy', *Amer. J. Psychiat.*, vol 125, no. 2, pp. 141–6.

BRYCE, F. O., HASLERUD, G. M., MITCHELL, G. D., WEINSTEIN, A. G., and NISWANDER, G. D. (1966), 'Problems in prediction of a schizophrenic population', *Arch. gen. Psychiat.*, vol. 15, pp. 140–43.

CAPLAN, G. (1964), *Principles of Preventive Psychiatry*, Basic Books,

CHAFETZ, M. E., and DEMONE, H. W. (1962), *Alcoholism and Society*, Oxford University Press.

CHODOFF, P. (1966), 'Effects of extreme coercive and oppressive forces: brainwashing and concentration camps', in S. Arieti (ed.), *American Handbook of Psychiatry*, vol. 3, Basic Books.

CLAUSEN, J. A., and KOHN, M. L. (1959), 'Relation of schizophrenia to the social structure of a small city', in B. Pasamanick (ed.), *Epidemiology of Mental Disorder*, no. 60, American Association for the Advancement of Science.

COHEN, B. M., and FAIRBANK, R. (1938a), 'Statistical contributions from the Eastern Health District of Baltimore. 1. General account of the 1933 mental hygiene survey of the Eastern Health District', *Amer. J. Psychiat.*, vol 94, no. 5, pp. 1153–61.

COHEN, B. M., and FAIRBANK, R. (1938b), 'Statistical contributions from the Eastern Health District of Baltimore. 2. Psychosis in the Eastern Health District in 1933', *Amer. J. Psychiat.*, vol. 94, no. 6, pp. 1377–95.

COHEN, B. M., FAIRBANK, R., and GREENE, E. (1939a), 'Statistical contributions from the Eastern Health District of Baltimore. 3. Personality disorder in the Eastern Health District in 1933', *Hum. Biol.*, vol. 11, no. 1, pp. 112–29.

COHEN, B. M., TIETZE, C., and GREENE, E. (1939b), 'Statistical contributions from the Mental Hygiene Study of the Eastern Health District of Baltimore. 4. Further studies of personality disorder in the Eastern Health District in 1933', *Hum. Biol.*, vol. 11, no. 4, pp. 485–512.

COOPER, B. (1961), 'Social class and prognosis in schizophrenia', pts 1 and 2, *Brit. J. prev. soc. Med.*, vol. 15, pp. 17, 31.

DUFF, D. F., and ARTHUR, R. J. (1966), 'Between two worlds: Filipinos in the US Navy', *Amer. J. Psychiat.*, vol. 123, no. 7, pp. 836–43.

DUMONT, M. (1968), *The Absurd Healer: Perspectives of A Community Psychiatrist*, Science House Inc.

EATON, J. W., and WEIL, R. J. (1955), *Culture and Mental Disorders*, Free Press.

EITINGER, L. (1964), *Concentration Camp Survivors in Norway and Israel*, Universitetsforlaget, Oslo.

EITINGER, L. (1969), 'Psychosomatic problems in concentration camp survivors', *J. psychosom. Res.*, vol. 13, no. 2, pp. 183–9.

FARIS, R. E. L., and DUNHAM, H. W. (1939), *Mental Disorders in Urban Areas: An Ecological Study of Schizophrenia and Other Psychoses*, Hafner.

FREUD, S. (1917), 'Mourning and melancholia', in *Collected Papers*, vol. 4, Basic Books and Hogarth Press.

GERARD, D. L., and HOUSTON, L. G. (1953), 'Family setting and the social ecology of schizophrenia', *Psychiat. Q.*, vol. 27, no. 1, pp. 90–101.

GOFFMAN, E. (1961), *Asylums*, Aldine; Penguin Books, 1968.

GOLDBERG, E. M., and MORRISON, F. S. (1963), 'Schizophrenia and social class', *Brit. J. Psychiat.*, vol. 109, no. 11, pp. 785–802.

GOLDHAMER, H., and MARSHALL, A. W. (1949), *Psychosis and Civilization: Two Studies in the Frequency of Mental Disease*, Free Press.

GRAD, J. C., and SAINSBURY, P. (1966), 'Problems of caring for the mentally ill at home', *Proc. Roy. Soc. Med.*, vol. 59, no. 1, pp. 21–5.

GRAVES, R. (1929), *Goodbye to All That*, Cassell; Penguin Books, 1960.

GREENWOOD, M. (1948), *Medical Statistics from Graunt to Farr*, Cambridge University Press.

GUNDERSON, E. K. E., ARTHUR, R. J., and RICHARDSON, J. W. (1968), 'Military status and mental illness', *Military Med.*, vol. 133, no. 7, pp. 543–9.

HALLIDAY, J. L. (1948), *Psychosocial Medicine*, Norton.

HARE, E. H. (1956), 'Family setting and the urban distribution of schizophrenia', *J. ment. Sci.*, vol. 102, no. 429, pp. 753–60.

HEMPEL, C. G. (1961), 'Morning session: introduction to problems of taxonomy', in J. Zubin (ed.), *Field Studies in the Mental Disorders*, Grune & Stratton.

HESTON, L. L., and DENNEY, D. (1968), 'Interactions between early life experience and biological factors in schizophrenia', *J. psychiat. Res.*, vol. 6, supp. 1, pp. 363–76.

HINKLE, L. E., JR, PLUMMER, N., and WHITNEY, L. H. (1961), 'The continuity of patterns of illness and the prediction of future health', *J. occup. Med.*, vol. 3, no. 9, pp. 417–23.

HOLLINGSHEAD, A. B., and REDLICH, F. C. (1955), 'Social stratification and psychiatric disorders', *Amer. soc. Rev.*, vol. 18, pp. 163–9.

HOLLINGSHEAD, A. B., and REDLICH, F. C. (1958), *Social Class and Mental Illness: A Community Study*, Wiley.

HOLMES, T., and RAHE, R. H. (1967), 'The social readjustment rating scale', *J. psycosom. Res.*, vol. 11, no. 2, pp. 213–18.

JACO, E. G. (1959), 'Mental health of the Spanish-American in Texas', in M. K. Opler (ed.), *Culture and Mental Health*, Macmillan Co.

JONES, M. (1953), *The Therapeutic Community*, Basic Books.

JONES, M. (1968), *Beyond the Therapeutic Community*, Yale University Press.

KARMEL, M. (1969), 'Total institution and self-mortification', *J. Health soc. Behav.*, vol. 10, no. 2, pp. 134–41.

KADUSHIN, C. (1964), 'Social class and the experience of ill-health', *Sociol. Inquiry*, vol. 34, pp. 67–80.

KENDELL, R. E. (1969), 'Discussion: the problems raised by cross-cultural studies', *Amer. J. Psychiat.*, vol. 125, no. 10 supp., pp. 41–3.

KRAMER, M. (1969), 'Cross-national study of diagnosis of the mental disorders: origin of the problem', *Amer. J. Psychiat.*, vol. 125, no. 10 supp., pp. 1–11.

KREITMAN, N. (1961), 'The reliability of psychiatric diagnosis', *J. ment. Sci.*, vol. 107, no. 450, pp. 876–86.

LEIGHTON, A. H. (1961), 'The Stirling County Study: some notes on concepts and methods', in P. H. Hoch and J. Zubin (eds.), *Comparative Epidemiology of the Mental Disorders*, Grune & Stratton.

LEIGHTON, A. H., and HUGHES, J. M. (1961), 'Cultures as a causative of mental disorder', *Milbank Memorial Fund Q.*, vol. 39, pp. 446–88.

LEIGHTON, A. H., LAMBO, T. A., HUGHES, C. C., LEIGHTON, D. C., MURPHY, J. M., and MACKLIN, D. B. (1963), *Psychiatric Disorder among the Yoruba*, Cornell University Press.

LEMKAU, P., TIETZE, C., and COOPER, M. (1943a), 'Mental-hygiene problems in an urban district, I', *Ment. Hyg.*, vol. 25, no. 4, pp. 624–46.

LEMKAU, P., TIETZE, C., and COOPER, M. (1943b), 'Mental-hygiene problems in an urban district, II', *Ment. Hyg.*, vol. 26, no. 1, pp. 100–119.

LEMKAU, P., TIETZE, C., and COOPER, M. (1943c), 'Mental-hygiene problems in an urban district, III', *Ment. Hyg.*, vol. 26, no. 2, pp. 275–88.

LEMKAU, P., TIETZE, C., and COOPER, M. (1943d), 'Mental-hygiene problems in an urban district, IV', *Ment. Hyg.*, vol. 27, no. 2, pp. 279–95.

LIDZ, T. (1963), *The Family and Human Adaptation*, International Universities Press.

LIN, T. Y. (1953), 'A study of the incidence of mental disorder in Chinese and other cultures', *Psychiat.*, vol. 16, no. 4, pp. 313–36.

LIN, T. Y., and STANDLEY, C. C. (1962), 'The scope of epidemiology in psychiatry', in *Public Health Papers*, no. 16, World Health Organization, Geneva.

LIN, T. Y. (1966), *Mental Disorders in Taiwan, Fifteen Years Later: A Preliminary Report*, Mental Health Unit, World Health Organization, pp. 1–17. Presented at the Conference on Mental Health in Asia and the Pacific, Honolulu, 29 March–1 April, 1966.

LYSTAD, M. H. (1957), 'Social mobility among selected groups of schizophrenic patients', *Amer. sociol. Rev.*, vol. 22, no. 3, pp. 288–92.

MALZBERG, B. (1962), 'Migration and mental disease among the white population of New York State 1949–1951', *Hum. Biol.*, vol. 34, pp. 89–98.

MENNINGER, K. (1968), *Vital Balance: The Life Process in Mental Health and Illness*, Viking Press.

MEYER, A. (1950–52), *Collected Papers*, 4 vols. ed. E. E. Winters, Johns Hopkins Press.

MISHLER, E. J., and SCOTCH, N. A. (1963), 'Sociocultural factors in the epidemiology of schizophrenia', *Internat. J. Psychiat.*, vol. 1, no. 2, pp. 258–305.

MORRIS, J. N. (1957), *Uses of Epidemiology*, Livingstone.

MURPHY, H. B. M., WITTKOWER, E. D., and CHANCE, N. A. (1964), 'Cross-cultural inquiry into the symptomatology of depression', *Transcult. psychiat. Res.*, vol. 1, no. 1, pp. 5–18.

MYERS, J. K., and BEAN, L. L. (1968), *A Decade Later: A Follow-Up of Social Class and Mental Illness*, Wiley.

NORRIS, V. (1959), *Mental Illness in London*, Oxford University Press.

ØDEGAARD, Ø. (1932), 'Emigration and insanity: a study of mental disease among Norwegian-born population in Minnesota', *Acta Psychiat. Neurol. Scand.*, supp. 4, pp. 1–206.

ØDEGÅRD, Ø. (1968), 'The pattern of discharge and readmission in Norwegian mental hospitals, 1936–1963', *Amer. J. Psychiat.*, vol. 125, no. 3, pp. 333–40.

OPLER, M. K. (1959), 'Cultural differences in mental disorders: an Italian and Irish contrast in the schizophrenias, USA', in M. K. Opler (ed.), *Culture and Mental Health*, Macmillan.

OSTWALD, P., and BITTNER, E. (1969), 'Life adjustment after severe persecution', *Amer. J. Psychiat.*, vol. 124, no. 10, pp. 1393–1400.

PICHOT, P. (1967), 'La nosologie psychiatrique et le diagnostic par ordinateur (Chroniques)', *La Presse Medicale*, vol. 75, no. 24, pp. 1269–74.

PIERCE, C. H. (1969), 'Violence and counterviolence: the need for a children's domestic exchange', *Amer. J. Orthopsychiat.*, vol. 39, no. 4, pp. 553–68.

PINDERHUGHES, C. A. (1969), 'Urban mental health issues' *Amer. J. Psychiat.*, vol. 125, no. 12, pp. 1721–2.

PLUNKETT, R. J., and GORDON, J. E. (1960), *Epidemiology and Mental Illness*, monograph series no. 6, Basic Books.

PUGH, T. F., and MACMAHON, B. (1962), *Epidemiological Findings in United States Mental Hospital Data*, Atlantic-Little, Brown.

RAHE, R. H. (1969), *Life Crisis and Health Change*, in P. R. A. May and J. R. Wittenborn (eds.), *Psychotropic Drug Response: Advances in Prediction*, Charles C. Thomas.

RAHE, R. H., ARTHUR, R. J., and GUNDERSON, E. K. E. (1971), 'Demographic and psychosocial factors in acute illness reporting' *J. chronic Diseases*.

RICHARDSON, B. W., and HAMPTON FROST, W. (eds.) (1936), *Snow on Cholera*, Oxford University Press.

RIESE, W. (1953), *The Conception of Disease, its History, its Versions, and its Nature*, Philosophical Library.

ROSANOFF, A. J. (1916), 'A survey of mental disorders in Nassau County, New York', *Psychiat. Bull.*, vol. 2, no. 2, p. 109.

RUSSELL, B. (1946), *A History of Western Philosophy*, Allen & Unwin; Simon & Schuster.

SABSHIN, M. (1969), 'The anti-community health "movement"', *Amer. J. Psychiat.*, vol. 125, no. 8, pp. 1005–12.

SAINSBURY, P. (1969), 'Social and community psychiatry', *Amer. J. Psychiat.*, vol. 125, no. 9, pp. 1226–31.

SASSOON, S. (1930), *Memoirs of an Infantry Officer*, Faber.

SCHERL, D. J., and ENGLISH, J. T. (1969), 'Community mental health and comprehensive health service programs for the poor', *Amer. J. Psychiat.*, vol. 125, no. 12, pp. 166–74.

SCHMALE, A. H., and ENGEL, G. L. (1967), 'The giving up–given up complex illustrated on film', *Arch. gen. Psychiat.*, vol. 17, pp. 135–45.

SHEPHERD, M. (1957), *A Study of the Major Psychoses in an English County*, Oxford University Press.

SIEGLER, M., and OSMOND, H. (1966), 'Models of madness', *Brit. J. Psychiat.*, vol. 112, no. 493, pp. 1193–203.

SIGERIST, H. E. (1958), *The Great Doctors*, Doubleday.

SROLE, L., LANGNER, T. S., MICHAEL, S. T., OPLER, M. K., and RENNIE, T. A. C. (1962), *Mental Health in the Metropolis: The Midtown Manhattan Study*, vol. 1, McGraw-Hill.

STANTON, A. H., and SCHWARTZ, M. S. (1954), *The Mental Hospital*, Basic Books.

STENGEL, E. (1964), *Suicide and Attempted Suicide*, Penguin Books.

SZASZ T. S. (1961), *The Myth of Mental Illness*, Harper & Row.

TURNER, R. J., and WAGENFELD, M. O. (1967), 'Occupational mobility and schizophrenia: an assessment of the social causation and social selection hypotheses', *Amer. sociol. Rev.*, vol. 32, no. 1, pp. 104–13.

WILMER, H. (1958), *Social Psychiatry in Action*, Charles C. Thomas.

WING, J. K. (1966a), 'Five-year outcome in early schizophrenia', *Proc. Roy. Soc. Med.*, vol. 59, p. 17.

WING, J. K. (1966b), 'The measurement of psychiatric diagnosis', *Proc. Roy. Soc. Med.*, vol. 59. pp. 1030–32.

WING, J. K. (1967), 'Social treatment, rehabilitation and management of schizophrenia', in A. Coppen (ed.) *Recent Developments in Schizophrenia*, Brit. J. Psychiat., monograph.

WING, J. K., BIRLEY, J. L. T., COOPER, J. E., GRAHAM, P., and ISAACS, A. D. (1967), 'Reliability of a procedure for measuring and classifying "present psychiatric state" ', *Brit. J. Psychiat.*, vol. 113, no. 498, pp. 499–515.

WYNNE, L., and SINGER, M. (1963), 'Thought disorders and family relations of schizophrenics. 2. A classification of forms of thinking', *Arch. gen. Psychiat.*, vol. 9, pp. 199–206.

ZEITLYN, B. B. (1967), 'The therapeutic community: fact or fantasy', *Brit. J. Psychiat.*, vol. 113, no. 503, pp. 1083–6.

ZUITHOFF, D. (1969), 'Community psychiatry and social action: the task of the social psychiatrist as a mental health consultant for the ministry of cultural affairs and social welfare, and the ministry of justice', *Scient. Proc. Summ. Form.* pp. 6–7, American Psychiatric Association.

Index

Abraham, K., 85
Ackland, H. W., 16
Adams, H. B., 26
Affective psychoses, 37
Alcoholism, cultural patterns, 110
Amok, psychiatric syndrome, Philippines, Indonesia, Malaya, 111–12
Arthur, R. J., 45, 47, 89, 108

Bean, L. L., 74
Bedlam Hospital (Hospital of St Mary of Bethlehem), London, 115
Berkeley, G., 16, 28
Bettelheim, B., 94
'Bilateral Project on Diagnosis of Mental Disorders', 107
Biochemical aspects of psychiatry, 155
Biosocial factors, effect of on mental health, Manhattan Study, 51–3
Bittner, E., 95
Bockoven, J. S., 41
Bridgman, P. W., 34
Brown, B. S., 144
Bryce, F. O., 42
Butterfield, H., 100

Camberwell register, 58–60
Cane Hill Hospital, London, 58

Cannon, W., 84
Caplan, G., 132
Carse, J., 135
Causes (projected) of prevalence of mental disorders, in lowest socio-economic classes, 80–81
Chafetz, M. E., 110
Chance, N. A., 105
Charcot, 26
Chichester, 135–9
Child-rearing patterns, interrelationship of psychosomatic disease incidence, 78–9
Chlorpromazine, introduction of, in psychiatric practice, 42
Chodoff, P., 94
Cholera
 epidemics, 16–17
 mode of communication of, 16–22, 147
Classification schemes, psychiatric, 35
Clausen, J. A., 78
Cohen, B. M., 50
Community Mental Health Centres, 134, 154
 evaluation of, 141–2
 Horsham, 134–5
 staffing and control of, 139–40
 'Worthing Experiment', 135–9

164 Index

Community psychiatry
 definition of, 130–31
 race problems, 143
 reorganization of society, 142–4
 summary, 153–4
Concentration camp syndrome, 94–6
Consultants, mental health in community organization, 140–44
Cooper, M., 50
Cooper, B., 82
Cornell Program in Social Psychiatry, 58

Decennial Survey, General Register Office, 64
Definitions, operational, for psychiatric disorders, 34–5
Demography, 12
 defined, 147
Demone, H. W., 110
Denney, D., 81
Diagnostic nomenclature, ten major categories, 36
Disease, Conceptual history, 23–5
Disease frequency
 prevalence, 14–15, 146–7
 incidence, 15, 148
Disease, homogenous distribution of, 64, 146–7
Duff, D. F., 108
Dumont, M., 142
Dunham, H. W., 75, 76

Eaton, J. W., 50, 103, 105
Echolalia, psychiatric syndrome, 111
Echopraxia, psychiatric syndrome, 111
Eitinger, L., 94

Engel, G. L., 85, 86
English, J. T., 142
Epidemiology
 defined, 12, 147
 seven uses of (J. N. Morris), 12–14
 Social Medicine Research Unit, London, 12
Esquirol, 39
Ethnopsychiatry, 101

Fairbank, R., 50
Fairhaven, Nova Scotia, 56
Family relationships and mental illness, 79–81
Faris, R. E. L., 75, 76
Farr, W., 63
Filipino recruits, US Navy, psychiatric admissions, 108–10
Freud, S., 26, 85
Frost, H., 16, 21

Galen, 23, 26
Genetic predisposition to mental illness, 80
Gerard, D. L., 78
'Giving up/given up' complex as precursor of mental illness, 85–6
Goffman, E., 119–22, 124
Goldberg, E. M., 76, 77, 82
Goldhamer, H., 44
Gordon, J. E., 60, 61
Grad, J. C., 135–7
Graunt, J., 15
Graves, R., 91
Graylingwell Hospital, Chichester, 134–9
Greene, E., 50
Greenwood, M., 38
Gunderson, E. K. E., 47, 90

Index

Halliday, J. L., 78
Hare, E. H., 82
Hawaii, State Mental Hospital, 152
Hempel, C. G., 34
Heston, L. L., 81
Hinkle, K. E., 11
Hippocrates, historic conception of disease, 15, 23
Hollingshead, A. B., 65, 70, 72, 74, 76, 77, 82, 149
Holmes, T., 87, 88
Hospitals, mental, admission and readmission rates, 42–8
  Goffman, 119–22
  mental factors affecting admissions, 39–42
  patients' length of stay, 41–3, 148–9
  Scandinavian countries, admission rates, 48
  social psychiatric history, 152–3
  Stanton, A. H., and Schwartz, M. S., 117–19
  Texas admission rates, 48–9
  US Navy, admission rates, 48
Houston, L. G., 78
Hughes, J. M., 114
Hume, D., 16, 22
Hutterite communities, culture and mental disorders, 103–5, 114, 152
Hysteria, mental illness and personal conduct, 26–7

Interview, and classification of patient's mental state, 32–3
Irish-Americans, study of cultural patterns and mental disease, 106–7

Italian-Americans, study of cultural patterns and mental disease, 106–7

Jaco, E. G., 48
Janet, P., 26
Johnson, S., 28
Jones, M., 125–7

Kadushin, C., 64
Karmel, M., 122
Kendall, R. E., 108
King's College Hospital, Southwark, 58
Knox, R., 28
Koch, R., 17
Kohn, M. L., 78
Koro syndrome in southern Chinese, Celebese and West Borneo, 112–13
Kramer, M., 45–6
Kreitman, N., 32

Lambo, T. A., 103
Langer, T. S., 51
Latah, psychiatric syndrome in Malaya, North Africa and northern Asia, 111
Lavallée, Nova Scotia, 56
Leighton, A. H., 53, 103, 114
Lemkau, P., 50
Lidz, T., 79
Lin, T. Y., 14, 50, 102, 151
Locke, J., 16
Lystad, M. H., 78

Malzberg, B., 98
MacMahon, B., 46
Manhattan, Midtown Manhattan Study, 51–3, 148
Manic-depressive disorders, UK and US, 108
Marshall, A. W., 44
Maudsley, H., 39

Maudsley Hospital, London, Social Psychiatric Research Unit, 58
Medical Research Council, Clinical Psychiatry Research Unit, Graylingwell Hospital, Chichester, 135
Menninger, K., 30
Mental illness, confrontations, challenges, 26–8, 146
Mental Treatment Act (1930), 130
Meyer, A., 84
Michael, S. T., 51
Midtown Manhattan Study, 51
Migration, influence upon mental disease, 98, 99
Mishler, E. J., 81
Morris, J. N., 12
Morrison, F. S., 76, 77, 82
Mortality rate, UK, 63
Murphy, H. B. M., 105
Myers, J. K., 74

National Institute of Mental Health, psychiatric registers, 58, 130
National Health Service, 130
New Hampshire Mental Hospital, admission rate, 42
New Haven, study of relationship between social class and mental illness, 65–6
Norris, V., 47
Nova Scotia, Sterling County Study, 53–8, 103, 148, 149

Ødegard, Ø., 48, 98
Old Manor Hospital, Salisbury, 137–9
Opler, N. K., 51, 106
Osmond, H., 29
Ostwald, P., 95

Paranoid personality, 36, 37
Paranoid schizophrenia in Filipino recruits, 109
Partial hospitalization
 day hospital, 132, 133
 emergency clinic, 132–3
 night hospital, 132–3
Pasma Sa Ugat and paranoid schizophrenia, 109
Patient council in therapeutic community, 126
Personality disorders
 paranoid personality, 36, 37
 schizoid personality, 36, 37
Petty, W., 15, 16
Pibloktoq, psychiatric syndrome in Polar Eskimo, 112
Pichot, P., 101
Pierce, C. H., 143
Pinderhughes, C. A., 143
Plato, concept of disease, 23
Plummer, N., 11
Plunkett, R. J., 60, 61
Prevalence of psychiatric impairment
 Manhattan Study (differential prevalence), 51–3
 Stirling County Study, 53–8
Preventive orientation of psychiatric disability
 primary prevention, 132–3
 secondary prevention, 132, 133
 tertiary prevention, 132, 133
Psychiatry
 biological basis of psychiatry, 155
 future directions, 155–6
 social psychiatry, 155
Psychopharmacology, 155

Psychophysical aspects of psychological perception scale, 88–9
Psychosomatic disorders, 38
Psychotherapeutic ideology, 141
Public attitudes towards mental illness, 155–6
Pugh, T. F., 46

Rahe, R., 87–9
Redlich, F. C., 65, 67, 68, 71, 72, 74, 76, 77, 82, 149
Rennie, T. A. C., 51
Richardson, B. W., 16, 21
Richardson, J. W., 47
Riese, W., 23
Rosanoff, A. J., 50
Russell, B., 28

Sabshin, M., 141
Sainsbury, P., 135, 136
St Christopher's Day Hospital, Horsham, 134
Salisbury, 'Worthing Experiment', 135–6
Sassoon, S., 91
Scherl, D. J., 142
Schizophrenia, 36, 37, 106–8, 152
 and social study, England and Wales, 76–7
 Camberwell Study, 58–60
Schmale, A. H., 85, 86
Schwartz, M. S., 117–19
Scotch, N. A., 81
Selye, H., 84
Shepherd, M., 47
Siegler, M., 29
Sigerist, H. E., 23
Singer, M., 79
Snow, J., 16, 17, 20–22, 147

Social class and mental illness, 15–16, 70, 73–4, 149
 categories of operations, 66
 controlled case study, 71–4
 follow-up study, 74
 hypothesis of, 65–6, 72–4
 interview schedule, 68–71
 mobility, social, 66, 75–8
 psychiatric treatment, 73–5
 social stratification, 70–75
Social classes, England and Wales, prevalence rates of disease, 64
Social disintegration, in relation to prevalence of psychiatric disorders, 56–8
Social mobility and mental illness, 66, 75–8
Social Psychiatric Research Unit, Maudsley Hospital, 58
Social psychiatry, 141–5
 education and training, 144
Sociocultural environment, operational definition, Stirling County Study, 53–4
Sociocultural factors, effects of Manhattan Study, 51–3
 Stirling County Study, 53
Sociotherapeutic ideology, 141
Somatotherapeutic ideology, 141
Srole, L., 51
Standley, C. C., 14
Stanton, A. H., 117–19
Stengel, E., 96
Stresses (social) and disease onset, 85–9, 150–51
 concentration camp, 94–6, 151
 war, 90–94
Suicide, influence of social events, 96–8, 151

Index

'Synedoche of success', 96
Szasz, T., 26–8, 34

Taiwan, Formosa, epidemiological study of psychiatric disorders, 102–3, 151
Therapeutic community, 125–7
  advocates of, 128–9
  criticisms of, 127–8
Tietze, C., 50
Transcultural psychiatry, 101, 113–14, 151–2
Tuke, S., 39
Turner, R. J., 78

Ufufuyana syndrome in Bantu of South Africa, 112

Virchow, R., 24
Von Rokitansky, C. F., 24
Voodoo syndromes, 113

Wagenfeld, M. O., 78
War, combat syndrome, 90–94

Weil, R. J., 50, 103, 105
Whitico or windigo, psychiatric syndrome, Hudson Bay area and Ogibwa Indians, 112
Whitney, L. H., 11
Wilmer, H., 125
Wing, J. K., 32, 58, 117
Wittkower, E. D., 105
Wolff, H. G., 84
World Health Organization International Classification of Disease (ICD–8), 36
'Worthing Experiment', Graylingwell Hospital, Chichester, 135–9
Wynne, L., 79

York Retreat-type hospitals, 115–16
Yoruba, Nigeria, study of psychiatric disorders, 110

Zeitlyn, B. B., 127
Zuithoff, D., 140

Penguin Science of Behaviour
Other titles available in this series:

Assessment in Clinical Psychology
C. E. Gathercole

Basic Statistics in Behavioural Research
A. E. Maxwell

Beginnings of Modern Psychology
W. M. O'Neil

Brain Damage and the Mind
Moyra Williams

Disorders of Memory and Learning
George A. Talland

Feedback and Human Behaviour
John Annett

Listening and Attention
Neville Moray

On the Experience of Time
Robert E. Ornstein

Pathology of Attention
Andrew McGhie

Personal Relationships in Psychological Disorders
Gordon R. Lowe

Psychometric Assessment of the Individual Child
R. Douglass Savage

Teachers and Teaching
A. Morrison and D. McIntyre

Vigilance and Attention
Jane F. Mackworth

Vigilance and Habituation
Jane F. Mackworth

Published simultaneously with this volume:

The Study of Twins
Peter Mittler

Many research workers are returning to twin studies as part of a renewed interest in the biology of human development. More specific questions are being asked, and more precise methods of analysis are being used. This book examines what is meant by 'the twin method' in psychology, and evaluates its basic assumptions. The main findings of twin research are summarized, with special reference to intelligence, personality, psychiatric disorders, and physical and biological aspects of development. The author also considers the contribution of twin studies not only to the 'nature – nurture' question, but also to basic problems in psychology and the developmental sciences.

Pattern Recognition
D. W. J. Corcoran

Pattern Recognition discusses psychological mechanisms involved in the process by which we identify and name a particular pattern from a whole class of patterns, such as a letter of the alphabet, a face or a voice. Taking as its main experimental paradigm the classification of multi-dimensional stimuli, the book considers the contribution of information theory to pattern perception, the part played by parallel and serial processing in recognition, the identification of patterns by computers, initial coding theories and the synthesis of whole patterns from their separate parts. The author sees pattern recognition as an analogue-to-digital conversion, with decision mechanisms in the system able to select an output at various levels of transformation of the input.

Penguin Modern Psychology Readings

Abnormal Psychology
Edited by Max Hamilton

Animal Problem Solving
Edited by A. J. Riopelle

Attitudes
Edited by Marie Jahoda and Neil Warren

Brain and Behaviour
1. Mood, States and Mind
2. Perception and Action
3. Memory Mechanisms
4. Adaptation
Edited by K. H. Pribram

Creativity
Edited by P. E. Vernon

Cross-Cultural Studies
Edited by D. R. Price-Williams

Decision Making
Edited by Ward Edwards and Amos Tversky

Experimental Psychology in Industry
Edited by D. H. Holding

Experiments in Visual Perception
Edited by M. D. Vernon

Freud and Psychology
Edited by S. G. M. Lee and Martin Herbert

Group Processes
Edited by Peter B. Smith

Intelligence and Ability
Edited by Stephen Wiseman

Language
Edited by R. C. Oldfield and J. C. Marshall

Leadership
Edited by C. A. Gibb

Motivation
Edited by Dalbir Bindra and Jane Stewart

Nature of Emotion
Edited by Magda B. Arnold

Perceptual Learning and Adaptation
Edited by P. C. Dodwell

Personality
Edited by Richard M. Lazarus and Edward M. Opton

Personality Assessment
Edited by Boris Semeonoff

Psychology and the Visual Arts
Edited by James Hogg

Skills
Edited by David Legge

Thinking and Reasoning
Edited by P. C. Watson and P. N. Johnson-Laird

Thought and Personality
Edited by Peter B. Warr

Verbal Learning and Memory
Edited by Leo Postman and Geoffrey Keppel

Volumes recently published in this series:

Creativity
Edited by P. E. Vernon

Creativity is a subject of great contemporary interest: how far, for example, can our educational systems promote or hinder the development of creative talents, either artistic or scientific?

This book covers a range and variety of work, both theoretical and applied, in creativity: studies of genius and of highly talented children, including the classical historical discussions by Galton and Terman; the nature of inspiration and of the production of original work in the arts and sciences, illustrated by introspective material by Mozart, Tchaikovsky, Stephen Spender and Henri Poincaré; the attempts of psychologists to measure creative talents by 'open-ended' or 'divergent thinking' tests; the personality characteristics of the creative individual; and the effect of education or special training on the development of creativity.

Freud and Psychology
Edited by S. G. M. Lee and Martin Herbert

Freud's theories have always been the subject of great dispute: this volume brings together some of the major contributions in that dispute in a courageous attempt to 'check up on Freud'. This is a critical survey of Freud's work on genetics, psychosexual development, defence mechanisms, such as projection, fixation, displacement and identification, and the unconscious.

Group Processes
Edited by Peter B. Smith

This book brings together recent research papers on small-group processes in the ground between the psychology of individuals and the wider study of sociology. The editor has favoured an open-system approach to group performance, presenting research on the part played by the individual in a group and work on the functioning of the small group in a wider social context. Thus, not only are the effects of personality variables and individual attitudes on roles considered, but also intergroup relations, and the influence of the environmental structure in which the group exists. Other sections deal with theoretical issues and structural models, as well as normative activity and behaviour change. Dr Smith draws attention to the wide range of application of concepts being developed in this field, to 'groups of students, managers, shop-floor workers, soldiers and nurses'.

Thought and Personality
Edited by Peter B. Warr

This collection of Readings demonstrates the increasing extent to which psychologists realize they must go beyond the study of observed behaviour and offer an account of the mental events involved in an individual's experience. Dr Warr shows how a new experimental and statistical rigour has been brought to contemporary 'introspectionism' in the study of cognitive style and structure. The book includes papers concerned with the much explored constructs of cognitive dogmatism and rigidity; with consistency in forming and differentiating categories; with the part played by the total organization of an individual's conceptual system in the formation of his attitudes; and with the application of these constructs to political and religious belief, and their effect on interpersonal attitudes. Finally, work on the characteristics of psychopathological thought, especially in schizophrenia, is described.